also by america's test kitchen

Desserts Illustrated

Vegan Cooking for Two

Modern Bistro

Fresh Pasta at Home

More Mediterranean

The Complete Plant-Based Cookbook

Cooking with Plant-Based Meat

Boards

The Savory Baker

The New Cooking School Cookbook:
Advanced Fundamentals

The New Cooking School Cookbook:
Fundamentals

The Complete Autumn and
Winter Cookbook

One-Hour Comfort

The Everyday Athlete Cookbook

Cook for Your Gut Health

Foolproof Fish

Five-Ingredient Dinners

The Ultimate Meal-Prep Cookbook

The Complete Salad Cookbook

The Chicken Bible

The Side Dish Bible

Meat Illustrated

Vegetables Illustrated

Bread Illustrated

Cooking for One

The Complete One Pot

How Can It Be Gluten-Free
Cookbook Collection

The Complete Summer Cookbook

Bowls

100 Techniques

Easy Everyday Keto

Everything Chocolate

The Perfect Cookie

The Perfect Pie

The Perfect Cake

How to Cocktail

Spiced

The Ultimate Burger

The New Essentials Cookbook

Dinner Illustrated

America's Test Kitchen Menu Cookbook

Cook's Illustrated Revolutionary Recipes

Tasting Italy: A Culinary Journey

Cooking at Home with Bridget and Julia

The Complete Mediterranean
Cookbook

The Complete Vegetarian Cookbook

The Complete Cooking for
Two Cookbook

The Complete Diabetes Cookbook

The Complete Slow Cooker

The Complete Make-Ahead Cookbook

Just Add Sauce

How to Braise Everything

How to Roast Everything

Nutritious Delicious

What Good Cooks Know

Cook's Science

The Science of Good Cooking

Master of the Grill

Kitchen Smarts

Kitchen Hacks

100 Recipes

The New Family Cookbook

The Cook's Illustrated Baking Book

The Cook's Illustrated Cookbook

The America's Test Kitchen Family
Baking Book

America's Test Kitchen Twentieth
Anniversary TV Show Cookbook

The Best of America's Test Kitchen
(2007–2023 Editions)

The Complete America's Test Kitchen
TV Show Cookbook 2001–2023

Healthy Air Fryer

Healthy and Delicious Instant Pot

Mediterranean Instant Pot

Cook It in Your Dutch Oven

Vegan for Everybody

Sous Vide for Everybody

Air Fryer Perfection

Toaster Oven Perfection

Multicooker Perfection

Food Processor Perfection

Pressure Cooker Perfection

Instant Pot Ace Blender Cookbook

Naturally Sweet

Foolproof Preserving

Paleo Perfected

The Best Mexican Recipes

Slow Cooker Revolution Volume 2:
The Easy-Prep Edition

Slow Cooker Revolution

The America's Test Kitchen
D.I.Y. Cookbook

**THE COOK'S ILLUSTRATED
ALL-TIME BEST SERIES**

All-Time Best Brunch

All-Time Best Dinners for Two

All-Time Best Sunday Suppers

All-Time Best Holiday Entertaining

All-Time Best Soups

COOK'S COUNTRY TITLES

Big Flavors from Italian America

One-Pan Wonders

Cook It in Cast Iron

Cook's Country Eats Local

The Complete Cook's Country
TV Show Cookbook

**FOR A FULL LISTING OF
ALL OUR BOOKS:**

CooksIllustrated.com

AmericasTestKitchen.com

praise for america's test kitchen titles

Selected as the Cookbook Award Winner of 2021 in the Health and Nutrition category
INTERNATIONAL ASSOCIATION OF CULINARY PROFESSIONALS (IACP) ON *THE COMPLETE PLANT-BASED COOKBOOK*

"An exhaustive but approachable primer for those looking for a 'flexible' diet. Chock-full of tips, you can dive into the science of plant-based cooking or just sit back and enjoy the 500 recipes."
MINNEAPOLIS STAR TRIBUNE* ON *THE COMPLETE PLANT-BASED COOKBOOK

"In this latest offering from the fertile minds at America's Test Kitchen the recipes focus on savory baked goods. Pizzas, flatbreads, crackers, and stuffed breads all shine here . . . Introductory essays for each recipe give background information and tips for making things come out perfectly."
BOOKLIST* (STARRED REVIEW) ON *THE SAVORY BAKER

"A mood board for one's food board is served up in this excellent guide . . . This has instant classic written all over it."
PUBLISHERS WEEKLY* (STARRED REVIEW) ON *BOARDS: STYLISH SPREADS FOR CASUAL GATHERINGS

"Reassuringly hefty and comprehensive, *The Complete Autumn and Winter Cookbook* by America's Test Kitchen has you covered with a seemingly endless array of seasonal fare . . . This overstuffed compendium is guaranteed to warm you from the inside out."
NPR ON *THE COMPLETE AUTUMN AND WINTER COOKBOOK*

"Here are the words just about any vegan would be happy to read: 'Why This Recipe Works.' Fans of America's Test Kitchen are used to seeing the phrase, and now it applies to the growing collection of plant-based creations in *Vegan for Everybody*."
THE WASHINGTON POST* ON *VEGAN FOR EVERYBODY

Selected as the Cookbook Award Winner of 2021 in the General category
INTERNATIONAL ASSOCIATION OF CULINARY PROFESSIONALS (IACP) ON *MEAT ILLUSTRATED*

"Another flawless entry in the America's Test Kitchen canon, *Bowls* guides readers of all culinary skill levels in composing one-bowl meals from a variety of cuisines."
BUZZFEED BOOKS ON *BOWLS*

Selected as the Cookbook Award Winner of 2021 in the Single Subject Category
INTERNATIONAL ASSOCIATION OF CULINARY PROFESSIONALS (IACP) ON *FOOLPROOF FISH*

"The book's depth, breadth, and practicality makes it a must-have for seafood lovers."
PUBLISHERS WEEKLY* (STARRED REVIEW) ON *FOOLPROOF FISH

"*The Perfect Cookie* . . . is, in a word, perfect. This is an important and substantial cookbook . . . If you love cookies, but have been a tad shy to bake on your own, all your fears will be dissipated. This is one book you can use for years with magnificently happy results."
HUFFPOST* ON *THE PERFECT COOKIE

"The book offers an impressive education for curious cake makers, new and experienced alike. A summation of 25 years of cake making at ATK, there are cakes for every taste."
THE WALL STREET JOURNAL* ON *THE PERFECT CAKE

"The go-to gift book for newlyweds, small families, or empty nesters."
ORLANDO SENTINEL* ON *THE COMPLETE COOKING FOR TWO COOKBOOK

"If you're one of the 30 million Americans with diabetes, *The Complete Diabetes Cookbook* by America's Test Kitchen belongs on your kitchen shelf."
PARADE.COM ON *THE COMPLETE DIABETES COOKBOOK*

"True to its name, this smart and endlessly enlightening cookbook is about as definitive as it's possible to get in the modern vegetarian realm."
MEN'S JOURNAL* ON *THE COMPLETE VEGETARIAN COOKBOOK

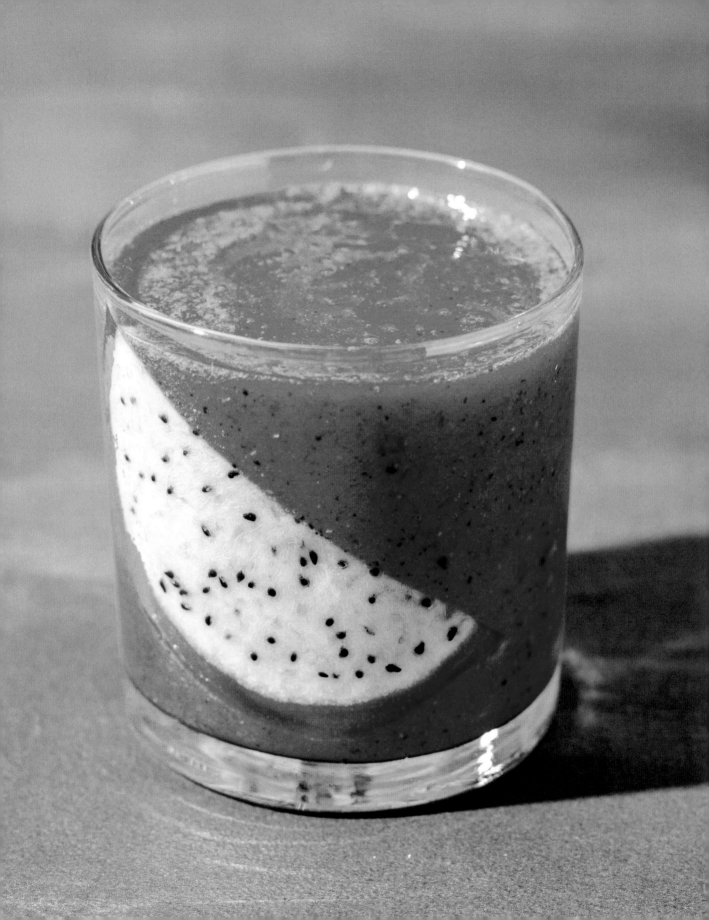

the complete guide to
healthy drinks

Powerhouse Ingredients • Endless Combinations

**Smoothies • Juices • Teas • Kombucha
Infused Waters • Broths and More**

AMERICA'S TEST KITCHEN

Library of Congress Cataloging-in-Publication Data

Names: America's Test Kitchen (Firm), author.
Title: The complete guide to healthy drinks : powerhouse ingredients, endless combinations : smoothies, juices, teas, kombucha, infused waters, broths, and more. / America's Test Kitchen.
Description: Boston, MA : America's Test Kitchen, [2023] | Includes index.
Identifiers: LCCN 2022039171 (print) | LCCN 2022039172 (ebook) | ISBN 9781954210202 (paperback) | ISBN 9781954210219 (ebook)
Subjects: LCSH: Beverages.
Classification: LCC TX815 .C66 2023 (print) | LCC TX815 (ebook) | DDC 641.2--dc23/eng/20220820
LC record available at https://lccn.loc.gov/2022039171
LC ebook record available at https://lccn.loc.gov/2022039172

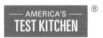

AMERICA'S TEST KITCHEN
21 Drydock Avenue, Boston, MA 02210

Printed in Canada
10 9 8 7 6 5 4 3 2 1

Distributed by Penguin Random House Publisher Services
Tel: 800.733.3000

Pictured on front cover (clockwise from left): **Rose Velvet Smoothie (page 63), Ginger Pomegranate Iced Black Tea (page 124), Cucumber Water with Lemon and Mint (page 162), Seriously Celery Juice (page 80), Kombucha (page 228), Cranberry Shrub Soda with Lime (page 212), Berry-Oat Smoothie (page 37), and Completely Carrot Juice (page 77)**

Pictured on back cover: **Cucumber and Kiwi Juice (page 90)**

Editorial Director, Books: **Adam Kowit**

Executive Food Editor: **Dan Zuccarello**

Deputy Food Editor: **Leah Colins**

Executive Managing Editor: **Debra Hudak**

Senior Editor: **Joseph Gitter**

Test Cooks: **Sãsha Coleman, Olivia Counter, Carmen Dongo, Jacqueline Gochenouer, Hannah Fenton, Eric Haessler, Hisham Hassam, José Maldonado, and Patricia Suarez**

Assistant Editor: **Emily Rahravan**

Kitchen Intern: **Olivia Goldstein**

Design Director: **Lindsey Timko Chandler**

Deputy Art Director: **Katie Barranger**

Associate Art Director: **Molly Gillespie**

Photography Director: **Julie Bozzo Cote**

Senior Photography Producer: **Meredith Mulcahy**

Senior Staff Photographers: **Steve Klise and Daniel J. van Ackere**

Staff Photographer: **Kevin White**

Additional Photography: **Joseph Keller and Carl Tremblay**

Food Styling: **Joy Howard, Sheila Jarnes, Catrine Kelty, Chantal Lambeth, Gina McCreadie, Kendra McNight, Ashley Moore, Christie Morrison, Marie Piraino, Elle Simone Scott, and Kendra Smith**

Thank you to Parachute Studios, Boston, Massachusetts, and Production Assistants: **Francesca Mignano and Tom Sinclair**

Project Manager, Publishing Operations: **Katie Kimmerer**

Senior Print Production Specialist: **Lauren Robbins**

Production and Imaging Coordinator: **Amanda Yong**

Production and Imaging Specialists: **Tricia Neumyer and Dennis Noble**

Copy Editor: **Karen Wise**

Proofreader: **Christine Corcoran Cox**

Indexer: **Elizabeth Parson**

Chief Creative Officer: **Jack Bishop**

Executive Editorial Directors: **Julia Collin Davison and Bridget Lancaster**

COVER
Photography: **Steve Klise (front); Kevin White (back)**
Food Styling: **Ashley Moore (front); Kendra Smith (back)**

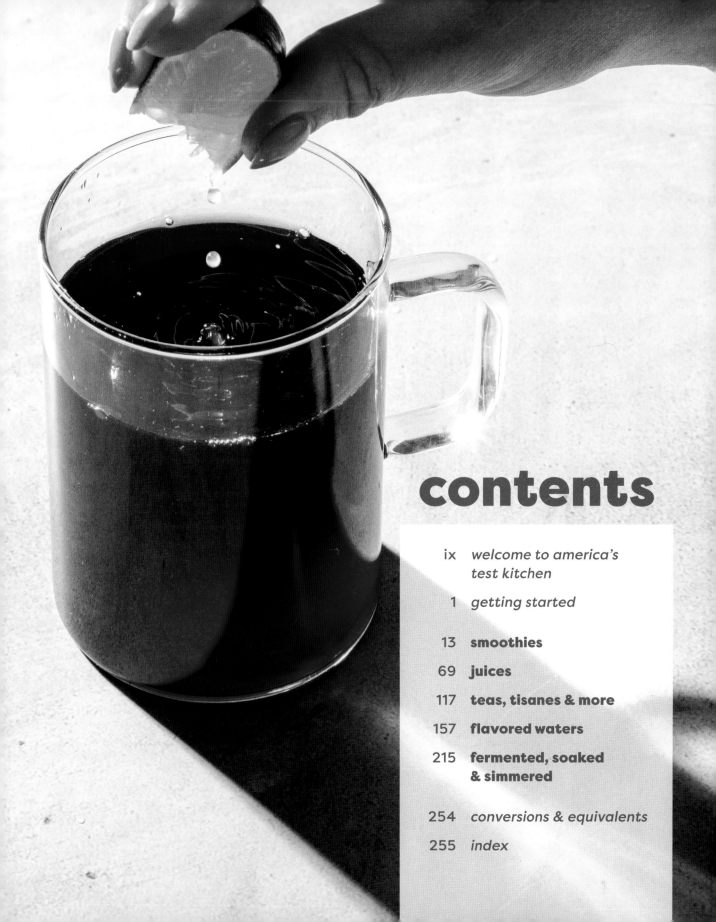

contents

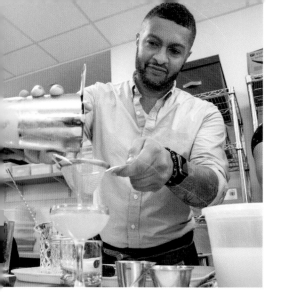
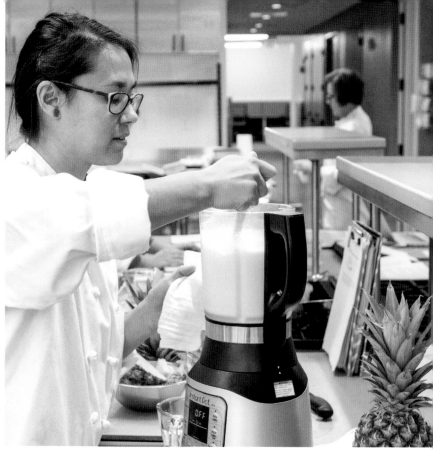
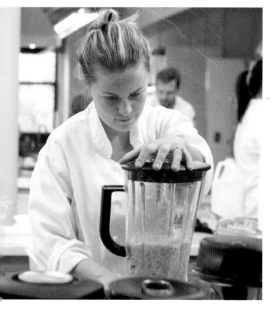
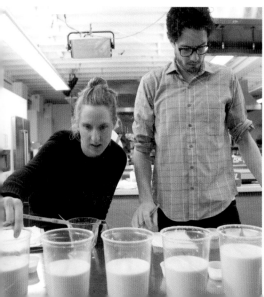
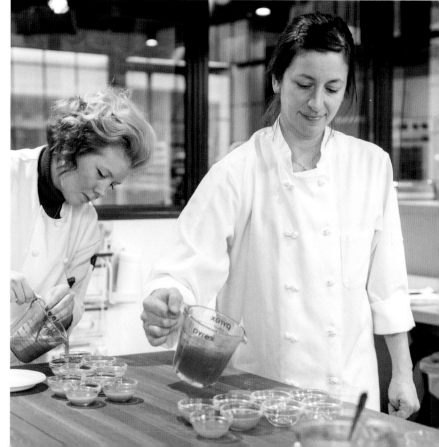

welcome to america's test kitchen

This book has been tested, written, and edited by the folks at America's Test Kitchen, where curious cooks become confident cooks. Located in Boston's Seaport District in the historic Innovation and Design Building, it features 15,000 square feet of kitchen space including multiple photography and video studios. It is the home of *Cook's Illustrated* magazine and *Cook's Country* magazine and is the workday destination for more than 60 test cooks, editors, and cookware specialists. Our mission is to empower and inspire confidence, community, and creativity in the kitchen.

We start the process of testing a recipe with a complete lack of preconceptions, which means that we accept no claim, no technique, and no recipe at face value. We simply assemble as many variations as possible, test a half-dozen of the most promising, and taste the results blind. We then construct our own recipe and continue to test it, varying ingredients, techniques, and cooking times until we reach a consensus. As we like to say in the test kitchen, "We make the mistakes so you don't have to." The result, we hope, is the best version of a particular recipe, but we realize that only you can be the final judge of our success (or failure). We use the same rigorous approach when we test equipment and taste ingredients.

All of this would not be possible without a belief that good cooking, much like good music, is based on a foundation of objective technique. Some people like spicy foods and others don't, but there is a right way to sauté, there is a best way to cook a pot roast, and there are measurable scientific principles involved in producing perfectly beaten, stable egg whites. Our ultimate goal is to investigate the fundamental principles of cooking to give you the techniques, tools, and ingredients you need to become a better cook. It is as simple as that.

To see what goes on behind the scenes at America's Test Kitchen, check out our social media channels for kitchen snapshots, exclusive content, video tips, and much more. You can watch us work (in our actual test kitchen) by tuning in to *America's Test Kitchen* or *Cook's Country* on public television or on our websites. Listen to *Proof*, *Mystery Recipe*, and *The Walk-In* (AmericasTestKitchen.com/podcasts) to hear engaging, complex stories about people and food. Want to hone your cooking skills or finally learn how to bake—with an America's Test Kitchen test cook? Enroll in one of our online cooking classes. And you can engage the next generation of home cooks with kid-tested recipes from America's Test Kitchen Kids.

Our community of home recipe testers provides valuable feedback on recipes under development by ensuring that they are foolproof. You can help us investigate the how and why behind successful recipes from your home kitchen. (Sign up at AmericasTestKitchen.com/recipe_testing.)

However you choose to visit us, we welcome you into our kitchen, where you can stand by our side as we test our way to the best recipes in America.

- facebook.com/AmericasTestKitchen
- instagram.com/TestKitchen
- youtube.com/AmericasTestKitchen
- tiktok.com/@TestKitchen
- twitter.com/TestKitchen
- pinterest.com/TestKitchen

AmericasTestKitchen.com
CooksIllustrated.com
CooksCountry.com
OnlineCookingSchool.com
AmericasTestKitchen.com/kids

getting started

When you think of healthy drinks, smoothies may be the first beverage that comes to mind. And while we love them, as you'll come to learn, there is a whole world of beneficial beverages beyond them. People reach for these drinks as a healthy option, but store-bought versions are often loaded with sugar and additional ingredients to keep them fresh. We believe that a great drink is made from a small blend of impactful ingredients, primarily consisting of fruits and vegetables, with minimal sweeteners.

You may be wondering "Why do I need a cookbook to make healthy drinks?" We did too. It seemed like those recipes wouldn't take much time to develop, but as we spent time in the kitchen, we discovered that there is a whole science to drink making and flavor blending that was more involved and nuanced than we expected. We were excited, and blown away. Test cooks lamented that they had missed a tasting when they heard how surprisingly delicious cabbage or celery juice or a particular tea blend was.

Because healthy drink making was new to us, we launched into it headfirst in the test kitchen, as is our practice. We tried every possible technique to perfect the recipes in the book so that everyone could easily prepare and drink their fruits and vegetables, soak their own nondairy milks, simmer protein-filled sipping broths, and blend their own teas. We tested dozens of different flavors and textures, even colors, to find just the right proportions of ingredients and the best ways to combine them.

We left no drink untested. We brought our rigorous approach and endless appetite for experimentation to the world of drinks to develop a complete range of healthful recipes. We dove deep into all categories of beverages and applied our science-based approach to make hydration healthful. We developed smoothies, juices, teas and tisanes, infused and flavored waters, and fermented, soaked, and simmered drinks. We also researched and created a number of recipes from different cultures, including cha manao from Thailand, tepache from Mexico, and haldhicha dudh from India.

Making your own drinks gives you more control over the ingredients you consume, can be more convenient, and even saves money over buying them premade. Plus, you get to expand your flavor horizons with all the unique tastes and textures that fruits, vegetables, herbs, and spices can bring to your drink world. This all-in-one guide and recipe book is your one stop for learning foolproof techniques and combinations so unique you may wonder how we thought of them: sweet corn and blueberries, chestnut and pear, and cherries and jicama, to name just a few.

The goal of this book was to develop drinks that are beneficial to you, that you will feel good about consuming, and that help you up your hydration game. The recipes deliciously fulfill that goal while also giving you the simple pleasure of preparing something really good to drink.

the drinks in this book

This book is complete in that we compiled an extensive range of drink types to cover every kind of healthy beverage, from morning juice to afternoon tea to evening hot chocolate. There is something for everyone, featuring endless flavor combinations. Join us on a drink-making exploration filled with fresh juices and smoothies, tea blends for relaxing alone or for sharing, refreshing waters for any time of day, fun fermented projects, simmered drinks and broths to warm you up, and bubbly spritzers to cool you down. You'll learn how to blend, brew, juice, infuse, ferment, spritz, soak, simmer, and everything in between. As you move through the book, you may notice that our yields change from chapter to chapter and sometimes from recipe to recipe. Each beverage category is unique, because while you may want a whole pitcher of fruit-infused water, the same cannot be said for smoothies and teas. The yields reflect a realistic serving size for that drink's shelf life, and for your equipment's capabilities.

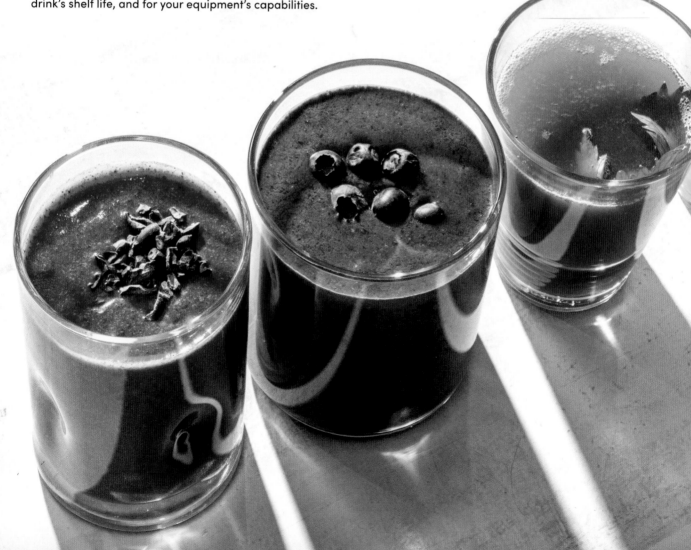

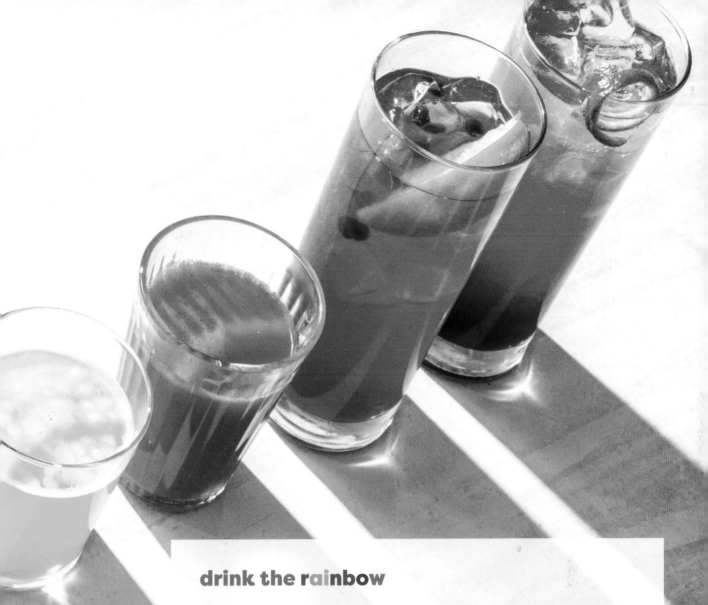

drink the rainbow

We made the nutritional guidelines for the recipes in this book as simple and realistic as possible to develop good-for-you drinks. We eliminated unnecessary ingredients and relied heavily on the natural goodness and flavor of fruits and vegetables, with supporting flavors coming from ingredients such as herbs, spices, nut butters, fruit juices, and milks. This book takes "Eat the rainbow" to heart because the most vibrantly colored fruits and vegetables are often the richest in vitamins, minerals, fiber, and antioxidants (which we all can use more of in our daily diet). The wide variety of drink types, temperatures, and textures you find here makes it easier to consume more healthful hydration. Sugar is sugar so we worked to avoid added sweeteners as much as possible and limited total sugar to below 20 grams per serving in all of our drinks. When we do employ it, we primarily stick to minimally processed sweeteners and smaller amounts. Where applicable, we also keep sodium amounts under control when venturing into the savory side.

why make your own drinks?

Although the prospect can seem daunting, making your own healthy drinks at home is easier than you think—not to mention easier on your body, free time, and wallet.

1 Have more control over the ingredients. When you make your own drinks, you know exactly what goes into them, and as a result, you know exactly what you'll get out of them nutritionally. Say goodbye to unpronounceable mystery ingredients and hello to good, clean drinks.

2 Get more interesting flavors with unique pairings. Just try our Sweet Corn and Blueberry Juice (page 92) or the sophisticated Bubbly Sage Cider (page 194). Additionally, we looked around the globe for inspiration to develop drinks such as tangy Mango Lassi (page 223) from India, refreshing Moroccan Mint Tea (page 141), and warming and nutritious Emoliente (page 144) from Peru.

3 Consume less sugar. Many drinks load up on sugar to impart sweetness and wake up dull flavors. Our drinks rely on fresh or frozen fruit and other ingredients to create flavorful and interesting profiles. We limited the amount of added refined sugar so that our drinks are healthier and more delicious and you can enjoy them more often.

4 Up your hydration game. Plain water can get boring, so this book provides healthful hydration options that you are more likely to drink. These liquids are tasty and easy to have on hand. Being hydrated keeps your body's basic functions afloat, so try an infused still or bubbly recipe (see pages 162–193) to make drinking water more enjoyable.

5 Spend less money. While buying a single drink can cost anywhere from $2 to $8, depending on the type, buying those same ingredients can bring your per-serving cost down tremendously, so your dollar goes further.

6 Make the classics. Make homemade versions of classic drinks for better-than-bottled V8 and Gatorade that taste more like their ingredients and less like preservatives. You don't have to give up what you like in the name of health—and in fact, you can improve upon them.

homemade versus store-bought

Take a look at how our recipes for homemade drinks compare to their store-bought counterparts. Our recipes are pared down to essential, nutritious, and delicious ingredients and eschew additives and other unnecessary items, to give you beverages that taste really good and are good for you.

✓ HOMEMADE PROS:

Short list of ingredients

No preservatives or additives

Less added sugar

Fresher-tasting ingredients

Loaded with fruits and vegetables

Endless exciting flavor combinations

Cost less

✗ STORE-BOUGHT CONS:

Long list of ingredients that may include preservatives

Often contain added sugars

Flavors don't taste as fresh

More processed, so lower nutritional benefits

Fewer flavor choices

Expensive

MAKE OUR DRINKS WORK FOR YOU

We know that everyone has different health needs, lifestyles, and dietary restrictions. This book puts flexibility at the forefront with the If You Don't Have feature of ingredient substitutions listed below each recipe. We swap out fresh for frozen, or swap in ingredients that may be available to you if you have something else on hand. You can make those trades with confidence, knowing that each recommendation was tested and approved by our test cooks. We also include options for different diets and offer dairy, nondairy, and plant-based alternatives when possible so that you don't have to miss out on any recipes. For ingredients that don't specify an amount, that means this is a direct 1-to-1 swap. If the quantity or prep instructions change, that is specified. If a specific variety for a fruit or vegetable isn't listed, that means any kind will work in the recipe.

SWEETENERS

In all of the recipes, we minimize added sugar and let the natural sweetness of the fruits and vegetables do the work. Occasionally, we turn to minimally processed sweeteners to help out: maple syrup, honey, agave, fruit juices, and dried fruits like dates and raisins.

simple syrup

We like to use less processed syrups like maple and honey, but in a pinch you can also make our easy no-cook simple syrup. It's ideal to sweeten all kinds of drinks (especially cold ones) since the sugar has already dissolved.

Combine equal parts sugar and warm tap water in a bowl, then whisk until sugar has dissolved. Let cool completely, about 10 minutes, then transfer to an airtight container. This syrup can be refrigerated for up to 1 month. Shake well before using.

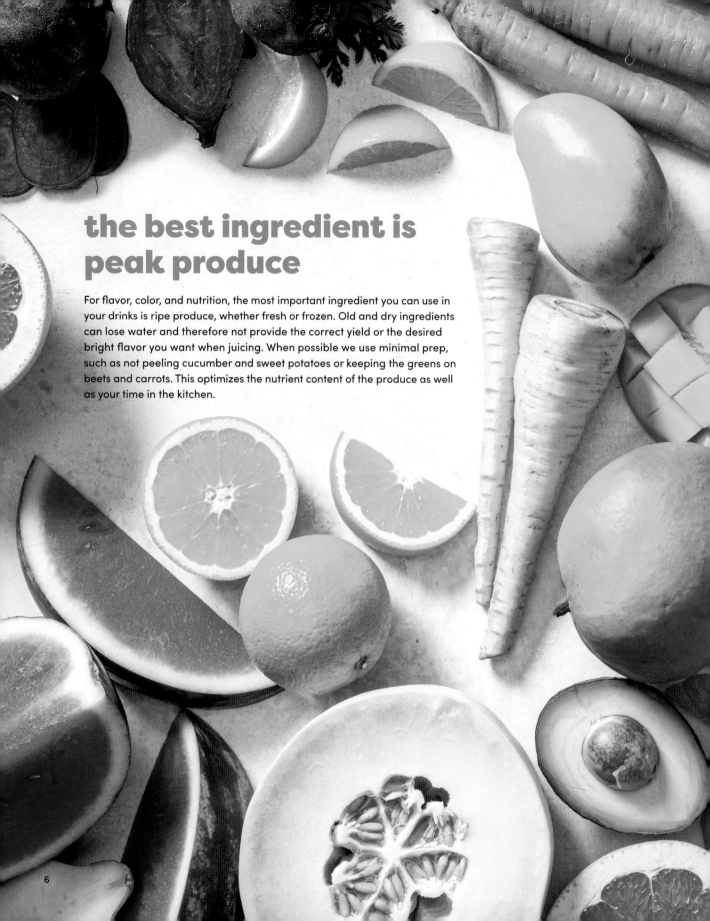

the best ingredient is peak produce

For flavor, color, and nutrition, the most important ingredient you can use in your drinks is ripe produce, whether fresh or frozen. Old and dry ingredients can lose water and therefore not provide the correct yield or the desired bright flavor you want when juicing. When possible we use minimal prep, such as not peeling cucumber and sweet potatoes or keeping the greens on beets and carrots. This optimizes the nutrient content of the produce as well as your time in the kitchen.

THE BUYER'S GUIDE TO FRESH PRODUCE

We call for produce in various ways throughout the book depending upon the chapter, but our approach to buying fresh fruits and vegetables remains the same. For peak ripeness and quality, we generally stick to these guidelines: Buy fruit when it starts to feel soft, and buy vegetables when they feel hard. This means that your fruit will approach ripeness within a few days and your vegetables have not turned limp or begun to lose water yet. Here are more specific things to look for when buying fresh produce to make our drinks.

avocados: Buy the small, rough-skinned Hass variety of avocados; they are creamy and less watery than other varieties. For a perfectly ripe avocado, look for one that is purple-black (not green) and yields slightly when gently squeezed.

beets: Healthy leaves are an easy-to-recognize sign of freshness when buying beets with stems and leaves attached. If buying roots only, make sure they are firm and the skin is smooth.

carrots: Buy fresh carrots with the greens attached for the best flavor. If buying bagged carrots, check that they are evenly sized and firm (they shouldn't bend). Do not buy extra-large carrots, which are often woody and bitter.

citrus: Look for fruit that feels heavy, with brightly colored skin that is free of blemishes. The fruit should not be overly firm and should yield when the skin is pressed (this indicates which fruit has the most juice).

dates: Although not technically "fresh," dates should look plump and juicy; skip over any that look withered or dry.

leafy greens: Leafy greens like baby spinach and kale are often sold prewashed in cellophane bags. Be sure to turn the bags over and inspect the greens closely. If you see moisture trapped in the bag or hints of blackened edges on the leaves, find a different bag.

mangos: Squeeze gently to judge ripeness. A ripe mango will give slightly, indicating soft flesh inside. Ripe mangos will also exude a sweet aroma at their stem ends.

melons: Look for heavy and firm fruit that has no indentations or soft spots. Smell the stem end—a ripe melon will have a slightly sweet fragrance. Cantaloupe should have corky veins that are visible over the rind, but the rind should not be green. It will continue to ripen at room temperature; once it's ripe, the rind will be golden yellow. A honeydew melon should be creamy white with a smooth surface. Once picked, it will not ripen further. Look for a watermelon that is firm and symmetrical with a yellow stem end. A ripe one will sound hollow when tapped.

pears: Choose pears that are ripe but firm; the flesh at the base of the stem should give slightly when gently pressed with a finger.

pineapples: Pineapples will not ripen further once picked, so purchase golden, fragrant fruit that gives slightly when pressed. You can also tug at a leaf in the center of the fruit: If the leaf releases with little effort, the pineapple is ripe.

storing produce: know your zones

We often think of a refrigerator as having a single temperature, but in fact every refrigerator has its own microclimates, and it is important to store ingredients properly within them (or outside the fridge completely).

IN THE PANTRY

The following produce should be kept at cool room temperature away from light to prolong shelf life: sweet potatoes, winter squash

IN THE FRONT OF THE FRIDGE

These items are sensitive to chilling injury and should be placed in the front of the fridge, where the temperatures tend to be higher: berries, corn on the cob, melons, oranges

ANYWHERE IN THE FRIDGE

These items are not prone to chilling injury and can be stored anywhere in the fridge (including its coldest zones), provided the temperature doesn't freeze them: apples, cherries, grapes

IN THE CRISPER DRAWER

These items do best in the humid environment of the crisper: beets, broccoli, cabbages, carrots, cauliflower, celery, chiles, cucumbers, herbs, leafy greens, lemons, lettuce, limes, peppers, summer squash, zucchini

ON THE COUNTER

These items are very sensitive to chilling injury and are subject to dehydration, internal browning, and/or pitting if stored in the refrigerator: apricots, avocados*, bananas*, eggplants, kiwis*, mangos, nectarines, papayas, peaches, pears, pineapples, tomatoes

Climacteric fruits continue to ripen once harvested. For this reason, they are often picked before fully ripe and are best left at room temperature (away from heat and direct sunlight) to mature. Once they've reached their peak ripeness, these fruits can be stored in the refrigerator to prevent overripening, but some discoloration may occur.

"WHAT ABOUT FROZEN?"

Having top-tier produce is key to getting the best, most delicious results, and sometimes frozen is the most logical way to get that great produce. Frozen fruits and vegetables are highly convenient and are picked and frozen at their peak ripeness. Whether there is a hard-to-find ingredient or out-of-season item, or we simply call for frozen because we want that icy texture and temperature in our drink, we use both fresh and frozen produce throughout this book to give you as much flexibility as possible in our recipes.

package produce properly

Appropriately storing your fresh produce can dramatically extend its shelf life. Be sure to keep vegetables either in their original packaging or in partially open plastic produce bags to help prevent moisture loss. Here is a list of more specific tips and techniques for keeping your ingredients fresh and ready to use.

beets: Beets with greens attached can be stored in the refrigerator in a loosely sealed zipper-lock bag for several days. If you remove the greens, beets will keep for one week, but save them for use in our Feel the Beet Juice with Beet Greens and Pear (page 78).

berries: Don't wash berries until you are going to use them. To store berries, place the berries in a zipper-lock bag or other container between layers of paper towels and refrigerate. Most berries freeze very well, but never wash berries before freezing, as they easily absorb excess water when rinsed. The water expands when frozen, causing the berry skins to rupture. Instead, spread them on a baking sheet or plate and freeze. After they are frozen solid, transfer the berries to a zipper-lock bag and freeze them for up to two months. A quick rinse helps jump-start the defrosting process.

broccoli: Store broccoli unrinsed in an open zipper-lock bag in the crisper drawer. It will keep for about one week. To revive limp broccoli, trim the stalk, stand it in 1 inch of water, and refrigerate it overnight.

cabbage: Keep cabbage loosely wrapped in plastic in the refrigerator for about four days. Remove the tough outer leaves before using.

carrots: For carrots with leaves, remove the greens before storing or the carrots will become limp. Keep the greens for use in our Completely Carrot Juice with Carrot Greens and Balsamic (page 77). Both bagged and fresh carrots will keep for several weeks.

cauliflower: Wrapped in plastic, cauliflower can be stored in the refrigerator for several days.

celery: Wrap celery in aluminum foil and store it in the refrigerator. It will keep for several weeks. Revive limp celery stalks by cutting off about 1 inch from both ends and submerging the stalks in a bowl of ice water for 30 minutes.

cucumbers: Cukes can be stored in the crisper drawer as is; the waxed coating most wholesalers apply will keep cucumbers fresh for at least one week. Unwaxed cucumbers can be stored in a loosely sealed zipper-lock bag for up to one week.

herbs: Store fresh herbs with roots attached at room temperature in a glass with water. Otherwise wrap herbs in damp paper towels and store in a zipper-lock bag in the crisper drawer.

leafy greens: Leafy greens (if bought bagged) should be stored in their original packaging, which is designed to keep them fresh. Flat-leaf spinach should be stored in a dry, open zipper-lock bag.

equipment to use

While working on this book, we tested our recipes on a wide range of equipment, from the recommended test kitchen winners listed here to a range of other models. The good news is that the recipes will work with whatever equipment you have.

BLENDERS

High-End Blender:
Vitamix 5200

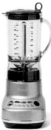

- Quiet and high-powered
- Simple, intuitive controls
- Narrow blender jar does not incorporate excess air during blending
- Watts: 1,491
- Capacity: 64 oz

Midpriced Blender:
Breville Fresh & Furious

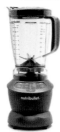

- Quiet and compact
- Automatically stops every 60 seconds, which makes tracking recipe stages very easy
- Watts: 1,300
- Capacity: 50 oz

Inexpensive Blender:
NutriBullet Full Size Blender

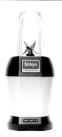

- Tall and lightweight
- Generous 8-cup capacity and a comfortable handle
- Very basic controls (low, medium, high, and pulse)
- Watts: 1,200
- Capacity: 64 oz

Personal Blender:
Ninja Nutri Ninja Pro

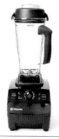

- Blades that angle both up and down for efficient blending
- Have to continuously hold down the pitcher to engage the motor
- Well-designed travel lid is comfortable to carry and drink from
- Watts: 900
- Capacity: 18 oz, 24 oz

JUICERS

Centrifugal Juicer:
Breville Juice Fountain Cold

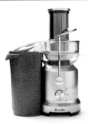

- Straightforward to assemble, with parts that fit together well
- Fast and produces smooth juices
- Contains debris fairly well and is easier to clean
- Feed tube diameter: 3 in

Masticating Juicer:
Omega Vertical Square
Low-Speed Juicer

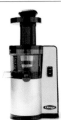

- Straightforward and enjoyable to use
- Relatively fast auger that chews through ingredients easily
- Easier to clean, especially with its included cleaning brush
- Feed tube diameter: 1.5 in

KETTLES

Electric: OXO Brew Cordless
Glass Electric Kettle

- Power switch lights up when it's activated
- Slow-open lid prevents accidental burns from steam and splashing water
- Has a removable filter in its spout
- Capacity: 17 to 60 oz

Best Buy: Cosori Original
Electric Glass Kettle

- Shuts off when the water reaches a boil
- Light-up power indicator and slow-open lid
- Lid conveniently opens when you press a button on the back of the handle
- Capacity: 16 to 56 oz

Stovetop: Chantal
Enamel-on-Steel Anniversary
Teakettle Collection

- Indicator whistle when boiling (whistle can be switched off)
- Works on all stove types
- Lightweight and easy to lift
- Capacity: 2 qt (64 oz)

SODA MAKER

SodaStream Terra

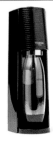

- Easy to use, with one large button on the top of the machine to press to desired level of carbonation
- Plastic water bottles connect to the machine easily and are dishwasher-safe
- Takes up fairly little counter space and is sturdy
- CO_2 source: gas canister

smoothies

smoothies 101

We went into the kitchen with a popular idea of what a smoothie is, but once we started testing, we realized it was more than bananas and strawberries with the occasional spinach thrown in. We wanted to create a wide range of smoothies with unique flavors, interesting textures, and unexpected ingredients. To up the nutritional content of our smoothies and to discover unheard-of combinations, we branched out to incorporate vegetables and found that smoothies are an ideal way to get more nutrients in your daily diet while enjoying the process.

blenders

WHAT TO USE AND WHAT TO KNOW

The blender that our test cooks used most frequently during recipe development for this book is our mid-priced winner, the **Breville Fresh & Furious**, as it is compact yet still powerful enough to process any smoothie efficiently. It automatically stops every 60 seconds, and its timer makes tracking recipe stages very easy. It is very easy to operate, while its price and wattage sits it in the middle of our overall range of winners, making it a great piece of equipment. We like the Breville because it is powerful enough to blend all our ingredients but not so powerful that the ingredients splatter up the sides of the blender jar. We prefer blenders with power over 750 watts, but our recipes will work in all blenders—just be sure to blend your drink until smooth and adjust the time as needed. For more information about our blender buying recommendations, see page 10.

personal blenders: If using a blender with a 3-cup (24-ounce) or less capacity, you will need to reduce each of the ingredients by half. Additionally, all ingredients will need to be added in reverse order as these blenders are typically inverted before blending.

> **"DO I NEED A VITAMIX?"**
>
> Blenders have a wide range of price tags, from $60 to almost $600, and it can feel as if you need a higher-powered one if you are a regular smoothie drinker. The fact of the matter is, any blender can be used to make a smoothie. The consistency of your drink is most important, so just be sure to blend until smooth (even if it is a longer time than called for in the recipe). So, while a Vitamix certainly doesn't hurt, you don't need one to make the smoothies in this book.

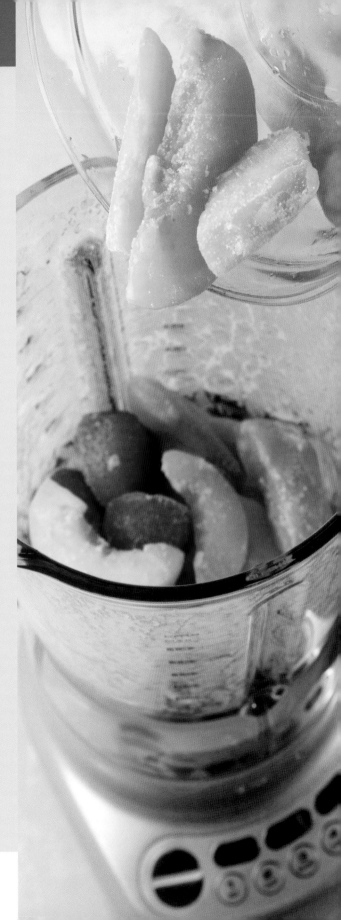

best blending techniques

ORDER IS VERY IMPORTANT

Our ingredient lists follow a specific order to create an effective vortex in the blender, which allows the ingredients to process quickly without the need for stopping, stirring, and starting up again. Solids and ice give the blade something to grip and get it turning, while liquid thins the ingredients so they can turn.

- Make sure to layer the solids into the blender first, so the blade can start breaking them down right away.

- Then add the ice to the blender, then the remaining solids, then liquids.

TECHNIQUE AND TIME MATTER FOR TEXTURE

We found that for the most effective blending, starting on low speed and slowly ramping up to high was the best. Increase the speed gradually, one power level at a time (whatever that looks like on your blender). This helps maintain the vortex without sloshing ingredients up the side of the blender, ensuring everything properly breaks down.

- Keep the blender running to maintain a strong vortex.

- Scrape down the blender jar as needed, with the blender turned off.

Our standard blending time is 1 minute, but sometimes more is necessary when there are highly fibrous veggies or lots of large pieces. However, too much blending can warm up the smoothie and overblend elements. Aim for a smooth, homogeneous texture with no fibrous or pulpy bits, and avoid bubbly aeration. Thickness will vary depending upon the ingredients.

the role of different ingredients

Some standout ingredients are worth highlighting because they have a myriad of benefits and ways in which they can enhance a smoothie, each adding their own unique factor to the equation of these recipes.

FLAVOR BASE AND NUTRIENT CONTENT

fresh fruit and vegetables: Gives the smoothie its dominant flavors and nutritious bulk. Vegetables play a milder supporting role to sweet fruit, adding great body without much sugar.

frozen fruit and vegetables: Same as fresh but with the added convenience of year-round availability.

FLAVOR MODIFIERS

fruit juices: Provide acidity and sweetness to brighten the overall flavor. Work to balance vegetable-heavy smoothies.

nut butters: Add richness, bulk, and savory, nutty flavor, while acting as a thickener and emulsifier. All varieties are delicious, some more distinctive than others (cashew butter was the least distinctive).

TEMPERATURE

frozen produce: Creates a chilled smoothie without ice.

ice: Adds chilled, temperature-controlled, aerated texture and light body.

THICK, CREAMY CONSISTENCY

banana: Contributes flavor subtle enough to balance other ingredients with mild sweetness.

avocado: Acts as an emulsifier that provides smooth texture and leaves the flavor mostly unchanged.

silken tofu: Gives a protein boost and acts as an emulsifier that provides smooth texture. Use in moderation to not overpower the flavor of the smoothie.

yogurt: Gives a protein boost with distinct, tangy flavor. Use in moderation to not overpower the flavor of the smoothie.

THINNER CONSISTENCY

water or milk: Thins the smoothie without impacting the overall flavor when used in moderation.

SMOOTHIE BOOSTERS

Some people opt to boost their smoothies with healthful add-ins, such as hemp seed hearts, flaxseeds, chia seeds, whey protein powder, and more. Note that these additions may change the taste and texture of your smoothie slightly. Check the recommended serving size on the product packaging for the amount you need to add.

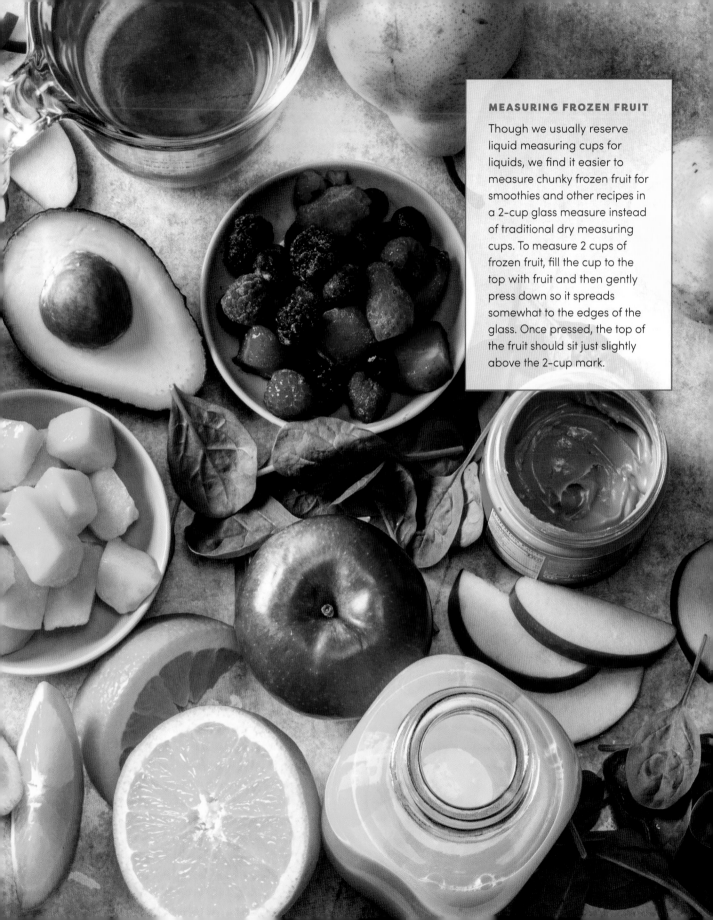

MEASURING FROZEN FRUIT

Though we usually reserve liquid measuring cups for liquids, we find it easier to measure chunky frozen fruit for smoothies and other recipes in a 2-cup glass measure instead of traditional dry measuring cups. To measure 2 cups of frozen fruit, fill the cup to the top with fruit and then gently press down so it spreads somewhat to the edges of the glass. Once pressed, the top of the fruit should sit just slightly above the 2-cup mark.

simplify your smoothie making

Smoothies are great at any point in your day, but you might not always have the time to whip them up immediately. Using the right storage container and having fruits and vegetables ready and in your fridge makes preparing a smoothie in minutes an achievable task anytime. We use these tips and tricks to have smoothies ready to make, or ready to enjoy, the next day.

smoothies on the go

ALWAYS RECOMBINE

Make your smoothie ahead of time so it's as simple as recombining ingredients just before drinking. All our blended smoothies can be refrigerated for up to 24 hours in the fridge. All you need to do to enjoy it the next day is stir vigorously before drinking.

MAKE IT IN A MASON JAR

By storing your smoothie in a Mason jar with a tight-fitting lid, you can easily shake it to recombine when drinking at a later date.

THE FREEZER IS YOUR FRIEND

Freeze blended smoothies in 1-ounce ice cube trays for up to 1 month. Simply pop out 8 to 12 smoothie cubes, thaw in a glass in the refrigerator overnight, and stir to recombine before drinking.

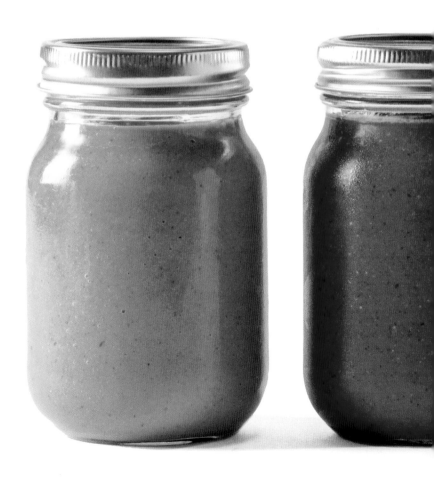

optimize your kitchen time

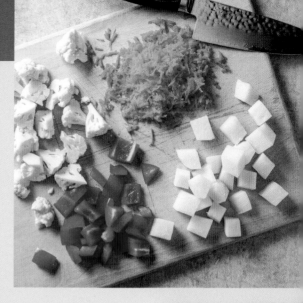

PREPARE VEGETABLES AHEAD
Chopping bigger vegetables, such as cauliflower, bell peppers, or jicama, right when you bring them home makes it that much easier to make your smoothie in a matter of minutes. You can also grate carrots in advance. Doing so can be time consuming, so we recommend grating them in bulk; then you just throw in the required amount when it comes time to blend your smoothie.

FREEZE RIPE BANANAS
Don't let your bananas go to waste. Cut peeled ripe bananas in half crosswise and store them flat in a zipper-lock bag in the freezer. Frozen bananas can be used interchangeably with room-temperature ones, but they do make the smoothie thicker and colder, and sometimes so thick that the blender won't catch the food and blend effectively. In this case you may need to add extra water, one tablespoon at a time, to allow the blender to catch, and you may need to increase the blender time by 30 seconds.

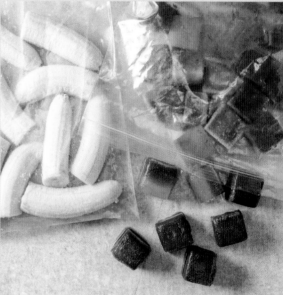

FREEZE THE GREENS
Have extra greens you want to save for future smoothies? For every 5 ounces of leafy greens (think baby spinach or kale), process with ¼ cup of water in a food processor, scraping down the sides of the bowl as needed until smooth, about 2 minutes. Transfer the finely chopped greens to ice cube trays and freeze, ready to pop into the blender for a green smoothie at a later date.

USE DIVIDED STORAGE CONTAINERS
For smoother smoothie pre-prep, you can store individual premeasured ingredients in a divided glass or plastic storage container, or set smaller containers within a larger one. Storing your ingredients together speeds up smoothie making, but keeping them separate is necessary for best blending practices.

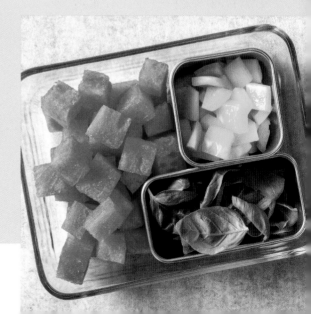

simple fruit smoothie

SERVES 2

- 2 cups frozen blueberries, raspberries, and/or strawberries
- 1 ripe banana, peeled and halved crosswise
- ¾ cup plain dairy or plant-based yogurt
- ¾ cup water, plus extra as needed

IF YOU DON'T HAVE

frozen berries: Use fresh berries and replace water with 1 cup ice.

why this combination works: This starter smoothie perfectly exemplifies the anatomy of a good smoothie, in both its combination of four simple ingredients and its straightforward method. We love berries for their inherent sweetness and tartness, but we worked to balance those flavors with the common smoothie additions of banana and yogurt. Both added a creamy element that made the drink smoother tasting and mellowed out any presence of berry seeds. Starting the blender on low speed helped minimize ingredients splashing up the sides of the jar, so after a quick scrape-down, we could use a higher speed to better emulsify the drink. Using water as our blending liquid let our ingredients take center stage while also thinning the smoothie enough for easy drinking. In addition to the master recipe, we offer variations, such as tropical-tasting mango-lime, that unite complementary flavors when you want a more curated combination.

In order listed, add all ingredients to blender and process on low speed until mixture is combined but still coarse in texture, about 10 seconds, scraping down sides of blender jar as needed. Gradually increase speed to high and process until completely smooth, about 1 minute. Adjust consistency with extra water as needed. Serve.

VARIATIONS

simple cherry-almond fruit smoothie
Substitute frozen sweet cherries for berries. Add 2 tablespoons creamy almond butter to blender following yogurt.

simple peach-vanilla fruit smoothie
Substitute frozen sliced peaches for berries. Add ¾ teaspoon vanilla extract.

simple mango-lime fruit smoothie
Substitute frozen mango chunks for berries. Add 1 teaspoon grated lime zest.

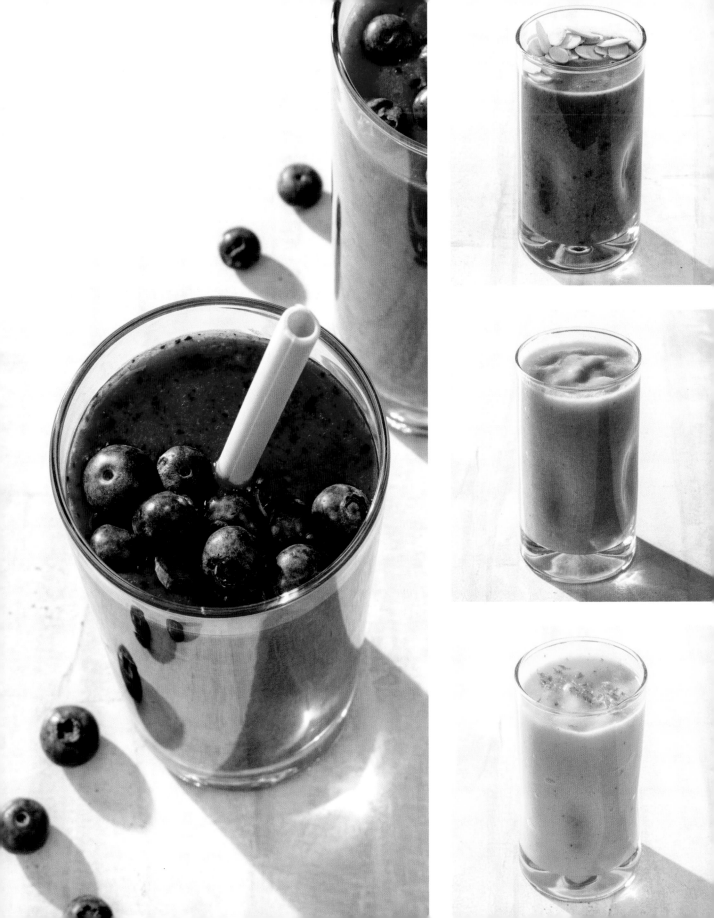

simple green smoothie

SERVES 2

- 1½ **cups baby kale**
- 1 **cup ice**
- 1 **ripe banana, peeled and halved crosswise**
- ½ **ripe avocado (optional)**
- ¾ **cup orange juice**
- ½ **cup water, plus extra as needed**

IF YOU DON'T HAVE

baby kale: Use 1½ cups stemmed and chopped mature green kale or baby spinach, or ½ cup frozen kale or frozen spinach.

orange juice: Use unsweetened apple juice.

why this combination works: This is our simplest vegetable smoothie, and it serves as a clean and green baseline that tastes sweetly vegetal. It's perfectly balanced, which means it tastes great by itself, but it can also take on other ingredients when you want to shake things up. For our green base, kale was the obvious choice because it is the king of green smoothies for its nutrient density and vegetal taste. When testing juices that we could add to the kale for some fruitiness, we discovered that both apple and orange juice worked with their mild sweetness and light acidity, but the orange had a more sharp and enticing flavor. Placing ice near the bottom of the blender helped add some aeration and coolness to the smoothie, while banana and avocado contributed a beautifully creamy, whipped texture to the drink (as well as added vitamins). You can omit the avocado; however, the smoothie will be less creamy.

In order listed, add all ingredients to blender and process on low speed until mixture is combined but still coarse in texture, about 10 seconds, scraping down sides of blender jar as needed. Gradually increase speed to high and process until completely smooth, about 1 minute. Adjust consistency with extra water as needed. Serve.

VARIATIONS

simple mango-pineapple green smoothie
Substitute pineapple juice for orange juice and ½ cup frozen mango chunks for avocado.

simple chocolate-orange green smoothie
Add 2 tablespoons cacao nibs or bittersweet chocolate chips and ¼ teaspoon grated orange zest to blender following avocado.

simple berry green smoothie
Substitute 1 cup frozen strawberries, raspberries, blackberries, and/or blueberries for avocado.

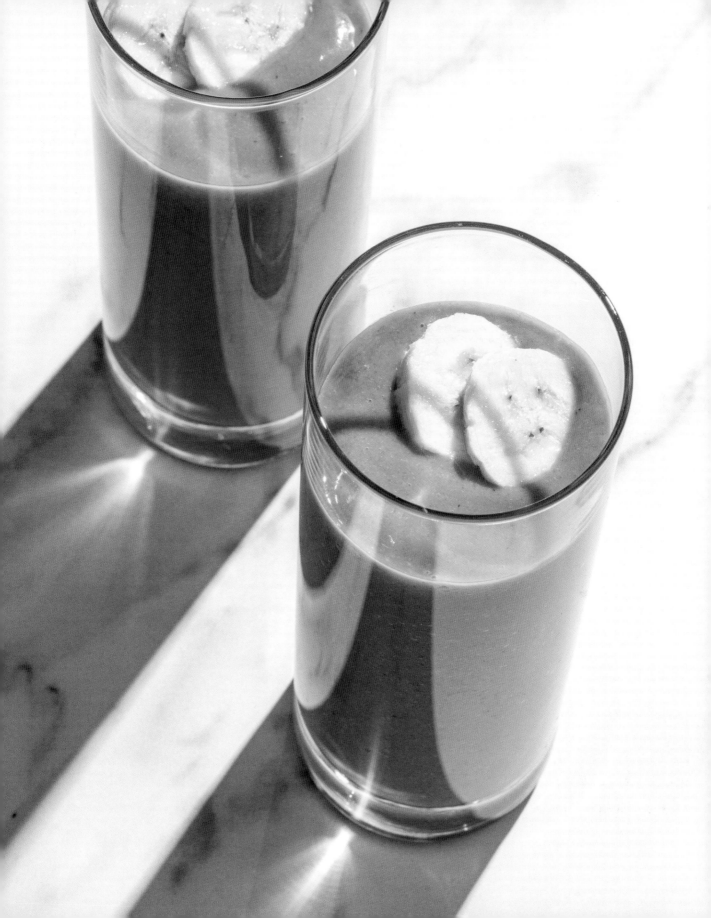

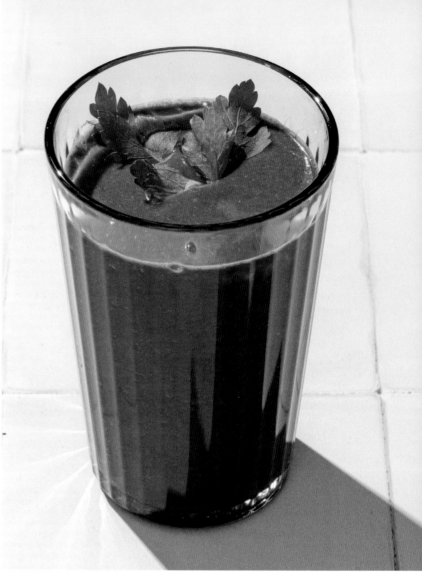
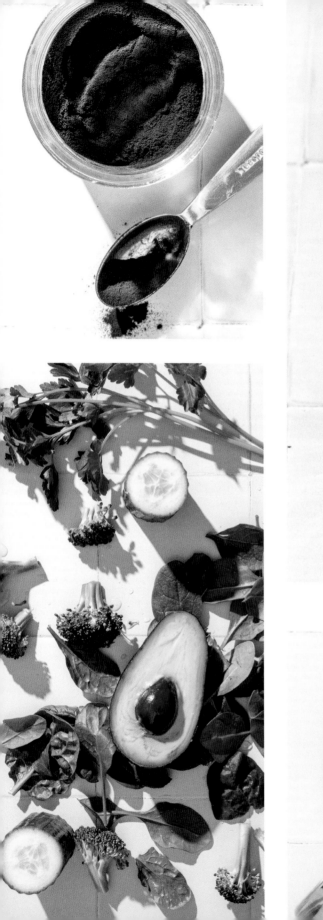
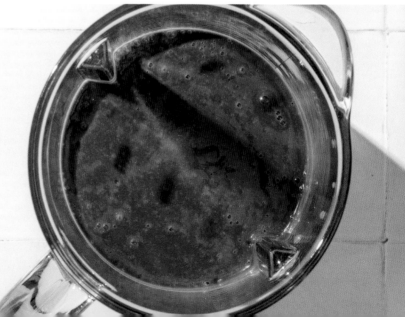

why this combination works: To some, a super greens smoothie is the epitome of healthy. To make sure our recipe delivered on that, we loaded ours with six beneficial greens. For a nutritious smoothie that was fresh and pleasantly vegetal, we carefully chose spinach and parsley, bitter (but not too bitter) greens with plenty of fiber; broccoli, which is actually quite sweet; refreshing cucumber; and avocado as an emulsifier and creamy thickener that held the smoothie together. Our final "green" came from the superfood spirulina, a plant-based blue-green algae high in omega-3 acids with strong antioxidant properties. Because all those greens can taste intense, we wanted a natural sweetener. Orange juice was too acidic against the greens, but unsweetened apple juice was a perfect neutral sweetener that balanced out the bitterness and rounded out the drink's flavor. Blending the ingredients with 2 cups of ice added some light aeration and broke up all the fibrous vegetables for a smooth, drinkable texture. Either blue or green spirulina can be used in this recipe, but blue spirulina will affect the color of your smoothie.

In order listed, add all ingredients to blender and process on low speed until mixture is combined but still coarse in texture, about 10 seconds, scraping down sides of blender jar as needed. Gradually increase speed to high and process until completely smooth, about 2 minutes. Adjust consistency with extra apple juice as needed. Serve.

super greens smoothie

SERVES 2

1 **cup baby spinach**

2 **cups ice**

4 **ounces cucumber, cut into 2-inch pieces (1 cup)**

3 **ounces broccoli florets, cut into 1-inch pieces (1 cup)**

½ **ripe avocado**

¼ **cup fresh parsley leaves**

2 **teaspoons spirulina (optional)**

1 **cup unsweetened apple juice, plus extra as needed**

IF YOU DON'T HAVE

spinach: Use 1 cup stemmed and chopped mature kale, baby kale, or baby arugula, or ⅓ cup frozen spinach or frozen kale.

broccoli: Use 3 ounces cauliflower florets, frozen cauliflower rice, chopped zucchini, or chopped carrots.

apple juice: Use apple cider.

matcha fauxba tea smoothie

SERVES 2

- 1½ cups baby spinach
- 1 cup ice
- 1 orange, peeled and quartered
- 1 very ripe Asian pear, peeled, quartered, and cored
- 4 ounces silken tofu
- 1–2 teaspoons matcha powder
- ¼ cup water, plus extra as needed
- ½ cup fresh or thawed frozen blueberries

IF YOU DON'T HAVE

Asian pear: Use Bosc, Anjou, or Bartlett pear.

why this combination works: Inspired by iconic boba tea with its chewy tapioca pearls, our burst of "fauxba" comes from thawed frozen blueberries, which have a similar look while contributing desirable nutrients. Boba is often enjoyed with a tea-based drink, so here we played with that expectation by adding 1 to 2 teaspoons of matcha powder to our smoothie. Matcha has a uniquely tannic flavor and provides a striking green hue in addition to some energizing caffeine. We kept things green with fiberful baby spinach but countered its slightly grassy flavor with a juicy orange and ripe pear. Our surprising ingredient here was silken tofu, which improved the overall texture of the beverage with a touch of soft creaminess. Plus, it offered a bit of plant-based protein. Placing the blueberries in the bottom of the glass before adding the smoothie on top is reminiscent of the boba-drinking experience, so this smoothie may best be enjoyed with a wide straw. Do not substitute soft or firm tofu. If storing, keep smoothie mixture and blueberries separately. Combine when ready to serve.

1. Add spinach, ice, orange, pear, tofu, matcha, and water to blender (in that order) and process on low speed until mixture is combined but still coarse in texture, about 10 seconds, scraping down sides of blender jar as needed. Gradually increase speed to high and process until completely smooth, about 90 seconds. Adjust consistency with extra water as needed.

2. Divide blueberries between 2 glasses and top with smoothie. Serve.

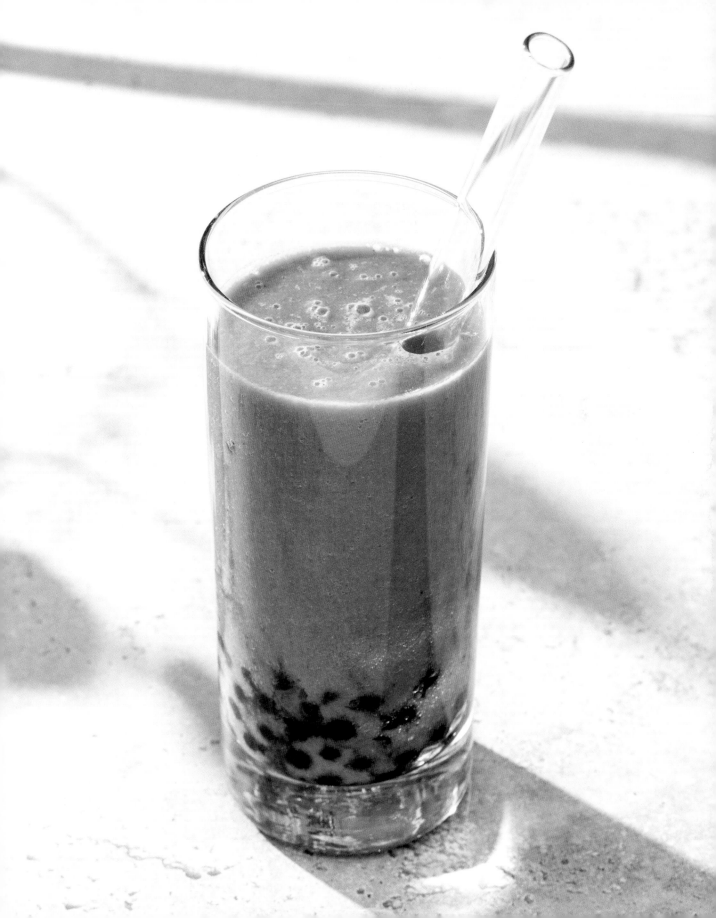

green apple pie smoothie

SERVES 2

2½ cups baby spinach

1¼ cups dairy or plant-based milk

⅓ cup walnuts, toasted
    and chopped

½ cup ice

1 apple, peeled, cored, halved,
   and cut into 1-inch pieces

½ teaspoon grated lemon zest

¼ teaspoon vanilla extract

⅛ teaspoon ground cinnamon

IF YOU DON'T HAVE

baby spinach: Use any baby green,
1½ cups chopped mature spinach, or
½ cup frozen spinach or frozen kale.

walnuts: Use pecans or cashews.

---

why this combination works: We approached this recipe with one goal in mind: Produce a spinach smoothie that made you want to drink your greens because it tasted like a classic baked apple dessert. A few extra steps in this recipe gave us a huge payoff in achieving that desired flavor outcome. For our apple element, we decided to stick with a fresh apple for its more suitable tart flavor, but peeling it first helped cut down on the mealy texture. Toasting the walnuts before adding them to the blender gave the smoothie a thickened texture and a nutty flavor that reminded us of a well-baked crust. During testing, we found that blending the spinach, walnuts, and milk first on high gave us a smooth paste to work with and created room in the blender jar for more ingredients after breaking down the 2½ cups of spinach. Finally, we enhanced that familiar apple-pie flavor by adding some zippy lemon zest, toasty-tasting vanilla extract, and a touch of warm cinnamon. We had the best success using McIntosh and Golden Delicious apples, as they blend well, but any variety will work.

1. Add spinach, milk, and walnuts to blender and process on high speed until smooth, about 1 minute.

2. Add ice, apple, lemon zest, vanilla, and cinnamon (in that order) and blend on low speed until mixture is combined but still coarse in texture, about 10 seconds. Gradually increase speed to high and process until completely smooth, about 90 seconds. Adjust consistency with extra milk as needed. Serve.

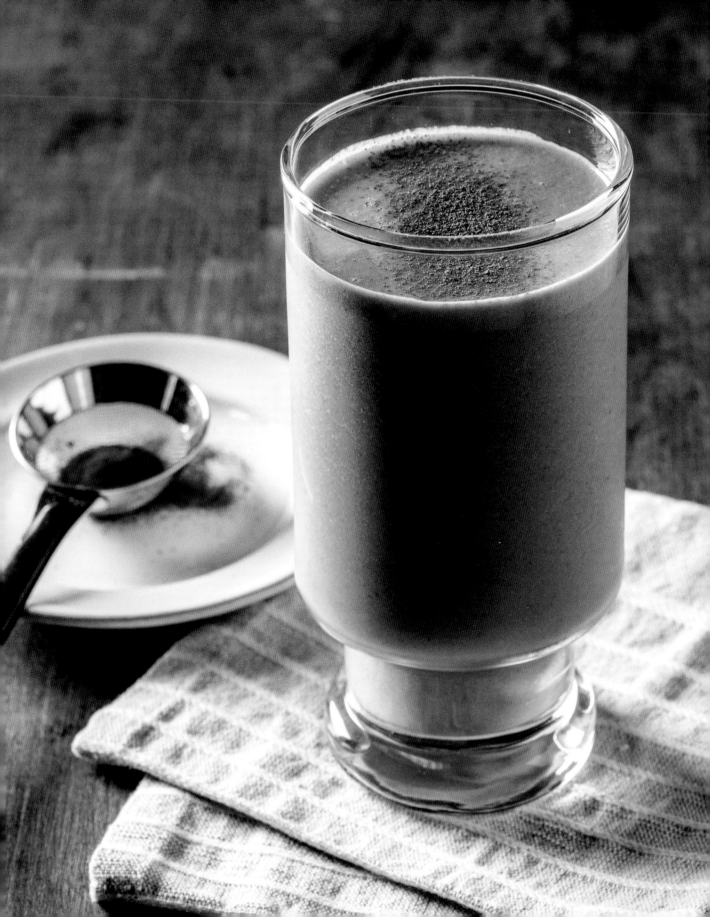

watermelon gazpacho smoothie

SERVES 2

½ **cup ice**

12 **ounces (1-inch) watermelon pieces (2 cups)**

1 **red bell pepper, halved, stemmed, and seeded**

1 **tomato, cored and halved**

¼ **cup fresh basil leaves**

1 **tablespoon extra-virgin olive oil**

½ **teaspoon red wine vinegar**

¼ **teaspoon pepper, plus extra for serving**

⅛ **teaspoon table salt**

IF YOU DON'T HAVE

red bell pepper: Use green, yellow, or orange bell pepper.

basil: Use cilantro or parsley.

red wine vinegar: Use white wine vinegar, balsamic vinegar, or sherry vinegar.

why this combination works: Whether made with fruits or vegetables, most smoothies taste on the sweeter side, but here we gave savory ingredients their time to shine. We took inspiration from the Andalusian cold soup gazpacho—typically made with tomato, bell pepper, oil, and vinegar—because tomato-based drinks are very popular and the soup itself combines many fresh ingredients. We employed watermelon here as our star ingredient because it has a similarly fruity profile to bell peppers without the bitterness. Additionally, the high water content of the watermelon worked to lighten and loosen the smoothie. We still seasoned with salt, pepper, red wine vinegar, and olive oil but simply used much less. The olive oil enhanced the smoothie by giving it rich and savory depth. We loved the addition of herby basil because it paired so nicely with the existing flavors and provided another fresh ingredient. Grinding extra pepper on top of the smoothie offers a savory aroma just before drinking that sets up your taste buds for the delightfully surprising drink to follow.

In order listed, add all ingredients to blender and process on low speed until mixture is combined but still coarse in texture, about 10 seconds, scraping down sides of blender jar as needed. Gradually increase speed to high and process until completely smooth, about 1 minute. Adjust consistency with water as needed. Sprinkle individual portions with extra pepper, if using, before serving.

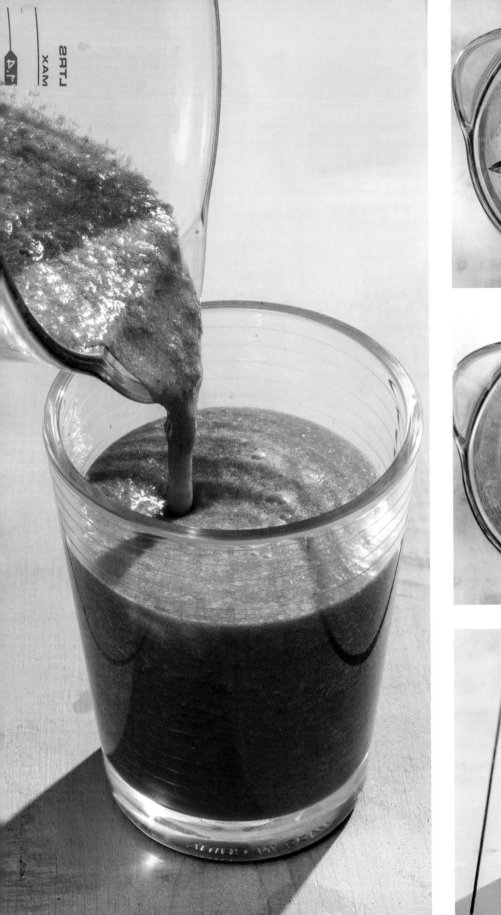
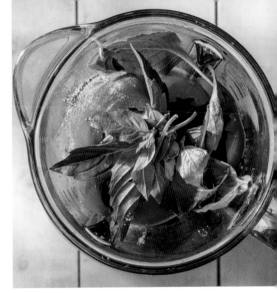
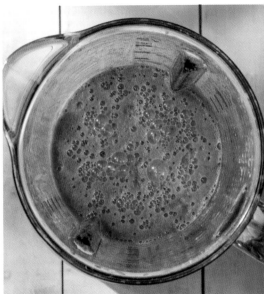
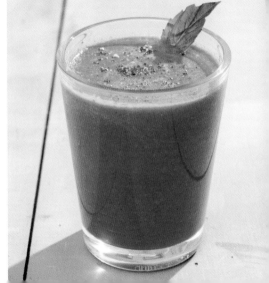

beets and berries smoothie

SERVES 2

8 **ounces peeled cooked beets, halved**

1½ **cups frozen strawberries**

1 **(1-inch) piece ginger, peeled and chopped**

1½ **cups water, plus extra as needed**

IF YOU DON'T HAVE

cooked beets: Use peeled and chopped raw beets.

frozen strawberries: Use frozen blueberries, raspberries, and/or blackberries. Fresh strawberries can also be used; replace water with 2 cups ice and increase processing time on high to 2 minutes.

why this combination works: Beets have a clean, earthy flavor with a bit of honey-like sweetness that we knew would pair nicely with berries for a uniquely delicious smoothie. Berries have a delectable flavor on their own, but here they accented the fruity undertones in the beets. The strawberries enhanced the sweetness in the beets and together made for a beautifully vibrant, red smoothie. Using frozen strawberries eliminated our need for added ice, but the smoothie still had a desirable chilled quality. We experimented with raw versus cooked beets but ultimately preferred the cooked ones because they had strong flavor and were softer, so they broke down nicely. For a pop of spice to complement this dynamic duo, we opted for ginger, which gave our smoothie a zippy note. Increasing the blending time cut down on the fibrous strands that can come from ginger, so the texture was nice and smooth. We had the best success using vacuum-sealed cooked beets; they are typically stored with other prepared fresh produce. Canned beets are also an option; be sure to purchase the unsalted variety and rinse them thoroughly before using.

In order listed, add all ingredients to blender and process on low speed until mixture is combined but still coarse in texture, about 10 seconds, scraping down sides of blender jar as needed. Gradually increase speed to high and process until completely smooth, about 90 seconds. Adjust consistency with extra water as needed. Serve.

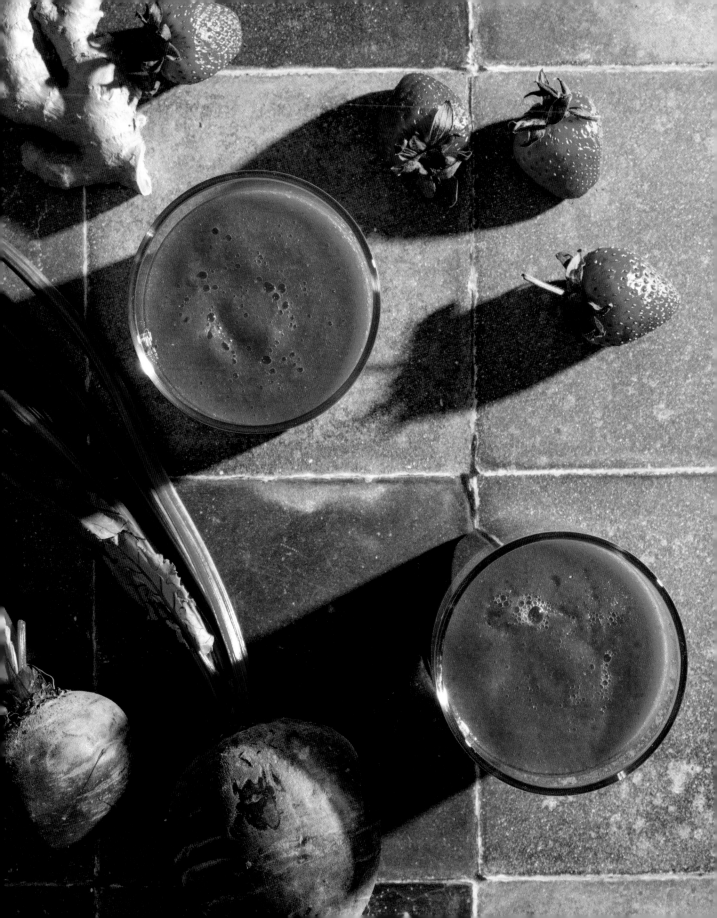

super açai smoothie

SERVES 2

1 **cup ice**

1 **(3.5-ounce) package frozen açai puree**

6 **ounces cauliflower florets, cut into 1-inch pieces (2 cups)**

1 **ripe banana, peeled and halved crosswise**

1 **cup pomegranate juice**

why this combination works: Açai is one of the most talked-about superfoods out there, so we took the popular açai bowl and turned it into a smoothie. Açai berries, which grow on palm trees in South America, are loaded with vitamins and antioxidants but have no sugar. When we tasted them raw, they were incredibly tart but intensely berryish, and that reminded us of that puckering flavor you find in pomegranate juice. This ended up being a perfect addition to our smoothie because we needed added liquid for blending but wanted to keep that sweet-tart, berry flavor. That pairing is potent (and not bulky enough for a full smoothie), so we balanced it with neutral cauliflower, which mellowed the flavors without diminishing their appeal. Our last ingredient was the ever-versatile banana, which contributed creamy sweetness that softened the sharp flavor of the berries for a profile that is sweet and fruity enough to enjoy a whole glass. Frozen açai puree is often sold in the freezer section with other fruits. Running the frozen package under warm water for 30 seconds makes it easier to remove the fruit from the packaging and blend it.

In order listed, add all ingredients to blender and process on low speed until mixture is combined but still coarse in texture, about 10 seconds, scraping down sides of blender jar as needed. Gradually increase speed to high and process until completely smooth, about 90 seconds. Adjust consistency with water as needed. Serve.

IF YOU DON'T HAVE

frozen açai puree: Use ½ cup frozen blueberries plus 1 tablespoon açai powder.

cauliflower florets: Use 6 ounces fresh or frozen cauliflower rice or broccoli florets.

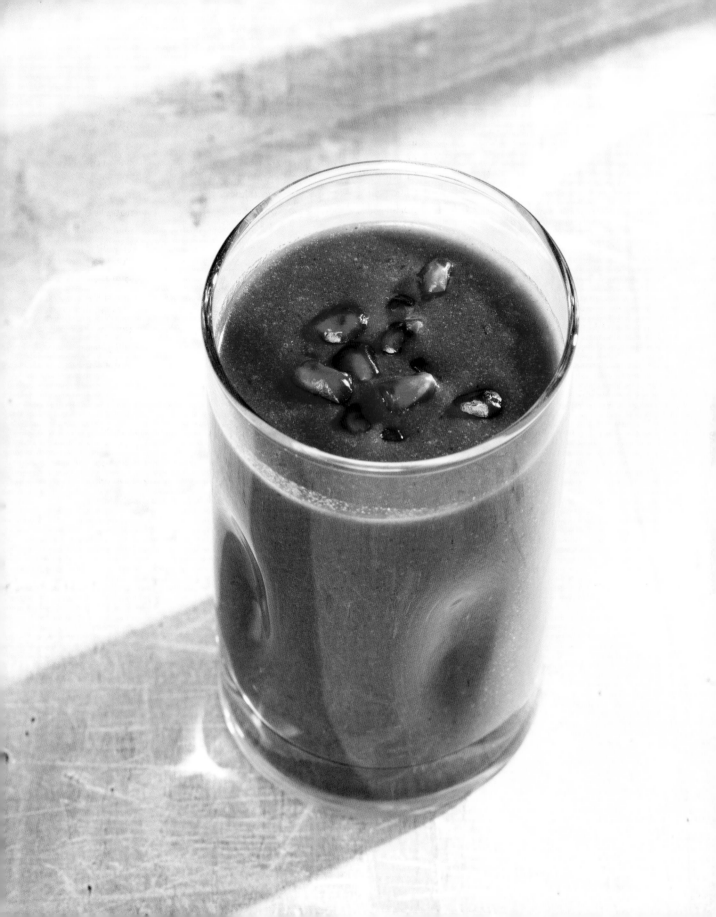

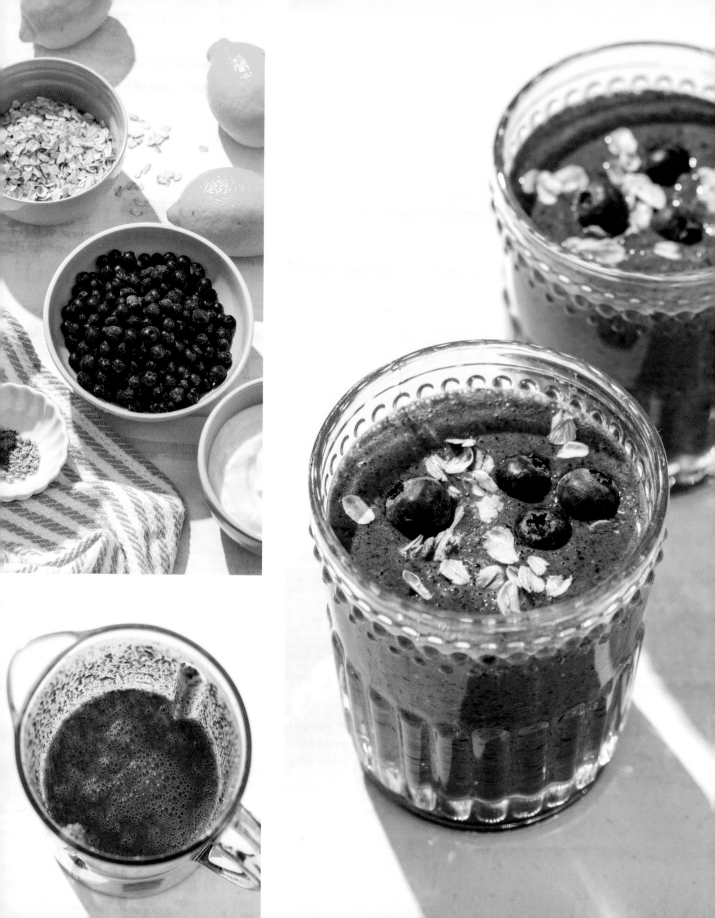

why this combination works: This smoothie feels like a treat because it evokes the comforting flavor of berry cobbler using naturally sweet ingredients (and some choice spices) while packing in fiber. To ensure an ideal mix of tart and sweet, we call for mixed berries. But despite the berries' star quality, it was the old-fashioned rolled oats that turned out to be the cornerstone of this smoothie, providing a thicker texture plus some good fiber. Though it may seem counterintuitive to toast the oats before blending them into a drink, the toasting helped create a nuttier, more intense flavor that leaned into that cobbler flavor profile. Adding yogurt to the mix made the smoothie creamier, and enhancing the smoothie with cinnamon, ginger, and bright lemon zest really emulated the baked dessert flavor that we aspired to. This recipe is flexible, so if you have a favorite cobbler, feel free to swap in whatever frozen berry you like best. Toast the oats in a dry skillet over medium heat until fragrant (about 2 minutes), then remove the skillet from the heat so the oats won't scorch. If storing overnight, thin the smoothie with additional water as needed because the oats will absorb liquid as they sit.

In order listed, add all ingredients to blender and process on low speed until mixture is combined but still coarse in texture, about 10 seconds, scraping down sides of blender jar as needed. Gradually increase speed to high and process until completely smooth, about 1 minute. Adjust consistency with water as needed. Serve.

berry-oat smoothie

SERVES 2

½ **cup old-fashioned rolled oats, toasted**

1¾ **cups frozen mixed berries**

½ **teaspoon grated lemon zest**

¼ **teaspoon ground cinnamon**

⅛ **teaspoon ground ginger**

½ **cup plain dairy or plant-based yogurt**

1 **cup water, plus extra as needed**

IF YOU DON'T HAVE

frozen mixed berries: Use 8 ounces frozen sweet cherries, strawberries, blueberries, and/or raspberries.

spicy mango smoothie

SERVES 2

1½ **cups frozen mango chunks**

1 **red bell pepper, stemmed, seeded, and chopped**

⅛ **teaspoon cayenne pepper**

1¼ **cups water, plus extra as needed**

Lime wedges for serving

why this combination works: Tropical fruit salad paired with spicy seasoning is a common snack in Mexico, so mangos, which have a uniquely tropical-floral flavor, made for a great jumping-off point. For a refreshingly zingy beverage, we combined the mango with a whole yellow bell pepper for its vegetal flavor and then kicked it up a notch with cayenne powder. While we loved the taste, we opted to switch to a red bell pepper for more vibrant color and slightly sweeter flavor. Using frozen mango chunks was a great way to keep our smoothie cold—and to find ripe mango year-round. For the blender blades to catch the chunks of mango, we knew we needed to use a lot of liquid but found orange juice to be overwhelming. Substituting water was a good solution, but we missed the acidity, so a hint of lime juice spritzed onto the smoothie just before serving provided that zip we desired against the sweet mango and rounded out the spicy-tropical flavor.

Add mango, bell pepper, cayenne, and water to blender and process on low speed until mixture is combined but still coarse in texture, about 10 seconds, scraping down sides of blender jar as needed. Gradually increase speed to high and process until completely smooth, about 90 seconds. Adjust consistency with extra water as needed. Serve with lime wedges.

IF YOU DON'T HAVE

red bell pepper: Use green, yellow, or orange bell pepper.

lime: Use lemon.

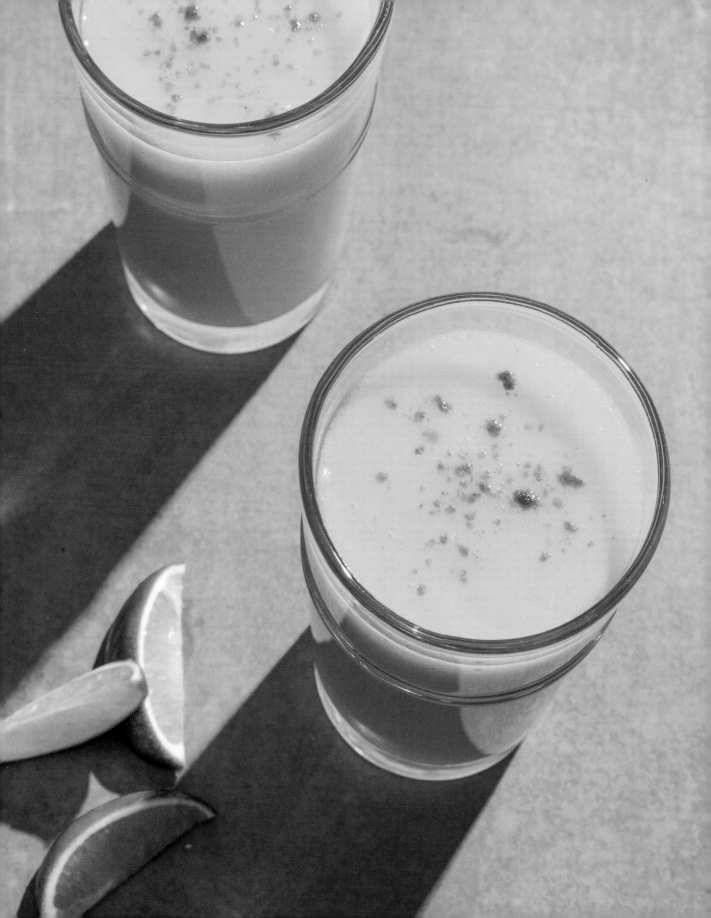

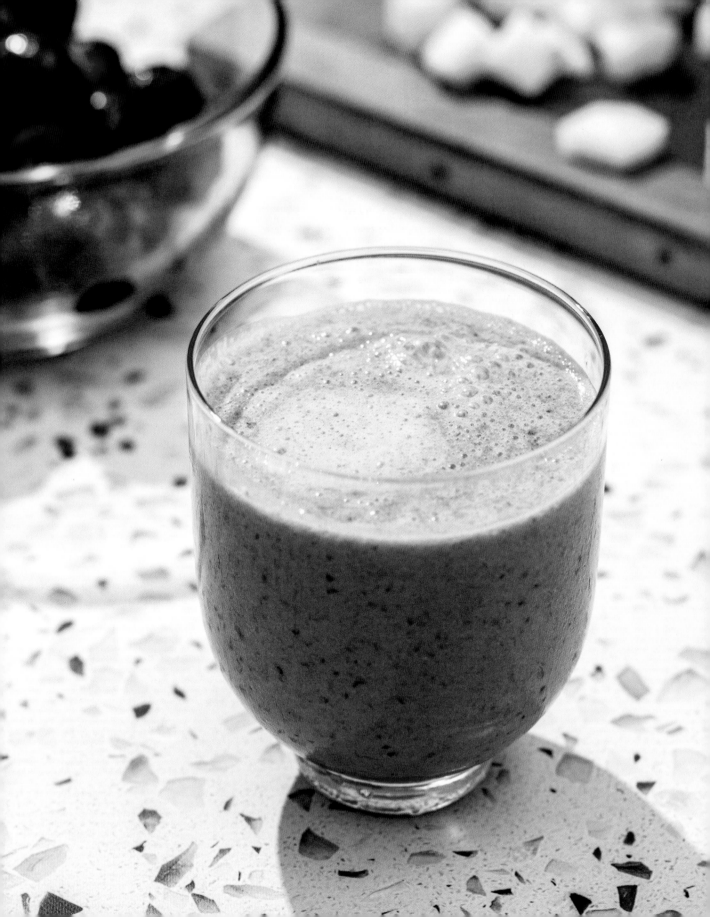

why this combination works: Cherries are one of the most popular fruits in the United States, so we wanted a smoothie that highlighted their beloved flavor while incorporating a vegetable for nutritious background. While cherries are decidedly seasonal, frozen cherries are always available, and they have the convenience of being pitted (so there's no need to make a mess for only 2 cups of them). Plus, they keep our final smoothie refreshingly cold. For increased body, we chose jicama, a starchy root vegetable that has been described as tasting like a cross between a potato and a pear. It gave neutral bulk, added fiber, and contributed minimal sugar, which was ideal as cherries themselves are higher in sugar than other berries. We were pleasantly surprised to discover how well the vegetable blended in, providing mild flavor but a refreshing crispness that really let the cherries shine through. We recommend peeling the jicama because otherwise you can end up with an unpleasant, waxy texture in your smoothie. We balanced the tartness of our cherry and jicama blend with creamy, tangy yogurt, which also gave us added protein and a smoother texture.

In order listed, add all ingredients to blender and process on low speed until mixture is combined but still coarse in texture, about 10 seconds, scraping down sides of blender jar as needed. Gradually increase speed to high and process until completely smooth, about 90 seconds. Adjust consistency with extra water as needed. Serve.

cherry-jicama smoothie

SERVES 2

- **2 cups frozen sweet cherries**
- **4 ounces jicama, peeled and chopped (1 cup)**
- **¾ cup plain dairy or plant-based yogurt**
- **1 cup water, plus extra as needed**

IF YOU DON'T HAVE

frozen sweet cherries: Use frozen strawberries, blueberries, and/or raspberries.

jicama: Use Asian, Bosc, or Bartlett pear, peeled, cored, and chopped.

minty melon smoothie

SERVES 2

1 **cup ice**

10 **ounces 1-inch honeydew pieces (2 cups)**

4 **ounces cucumber, cut into 2-inch pieces (1 cup)**

¼ **cup fresh mint leaves**

¾ **cup plain dairy or plant-based yogurt**

½ **cup water, plus extra as needed**

IF YOU DON'T HAVE

honeydew: Use cantaloupe.

mint: Use basil.

why this combination works: Taking inspiration from agua frescas and luxurious-tasting infused waters (pages 162–176), we translated their refreshing qualities into a thirst-quenching smoothie. We knew we wanted to include cucumber because of its subtle flavor and additional liquid thanks to its high water content. When considering other ingredients, we remembered the South American combination of melon and mint. Ripe honeydew melon blended with the crisp cucumber for a hydrating and slightly sweet flavor profile, while fresh mint leaves (though small in quantity) contributed a stimulating taste that accented the sweet melon and enhanced the refreshing cucumber. Thanks to the cucumber liquid, we needed only a small amount of additional water to get this smoothie mixing in the blender to our desired texture. Adding yogurt and ice created a more cohesive and cooling base for the flavors to meld into an invigorating drink.

In order listed, add all ingredients to blender and process on low speed until mixture is combined but still coarse in texture, about 10 seconds, scraping down sides of blender jar as needed. Gradually increase speed to high and process until completely smooth, about 1 minute. Adjust consistency with extra water as needed. Serve.

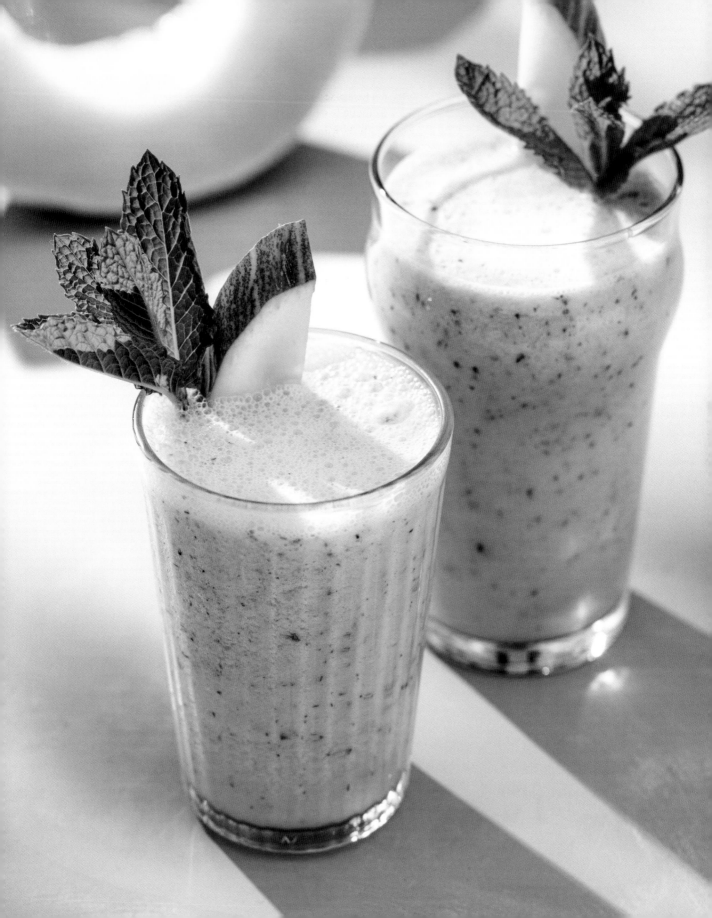

orange creamsicle smoothie

SERVES 2

- 1 **cup ice**

- 1 **orange, peeled and quartered**

- 1 **ripe banana, peeled and halved crosswise**

- 1 **large carrot, peeled and shredded**

- ¾ **cup plain dairy or plant-based yogurt**

- ¼ **cup water, plus extra as needed**

- ½ **teaspoon vanilla extract**

IF YOU DON'T HAVE

orange: Use 1 blood orange or 2 clementines.

why this combination works: The Creamsicle Bar is an ice-cream truck staple and childhood favorite, so we boosted that indulgence with nourishing ingredients. Oranges are the most popular citrus fruit and loaded with vitamin C, while a carrot delivered some sweetness, bulk, nutrients, and that distinctive orange hue. Orange juice can be on the sour side, so while it gave us extra orange flavor and much-needed liquid, we mellowed it with creamy components that also worked to emulate our inspiration. Mixing in yogurt and a banana greatly enhanced the overall velvety texture of our smoothie and provided milky sweetness that melded with the orange. A touch of vanilla extract helped balance out the tang of the yogurt and bring another hint of sweetness, but without the sugar. Thinning the mixture with water created the ideal thickness so the final smoothie had body while still being sweet and sippable.

In order listed, add all ingredients to blender and process on low speed until mixture is combined but still coarse in texture, about 10 seconds, scraping down sides of blender jar as needed. Gradually increase speed to high and process until completely smooth, about 2 minutes. Adjust consistency with extra water as needed. Serve.

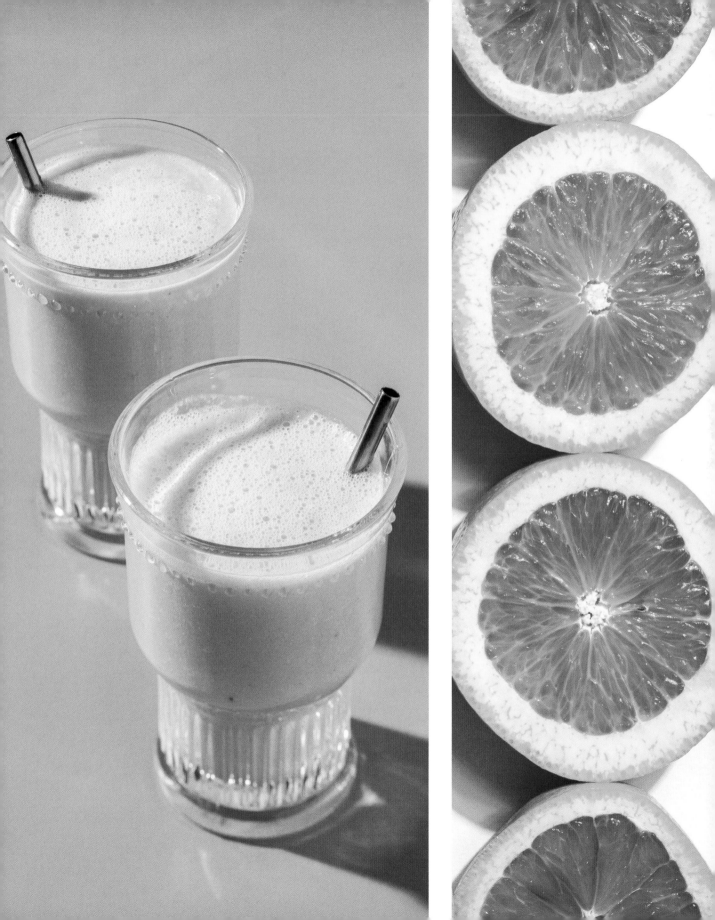

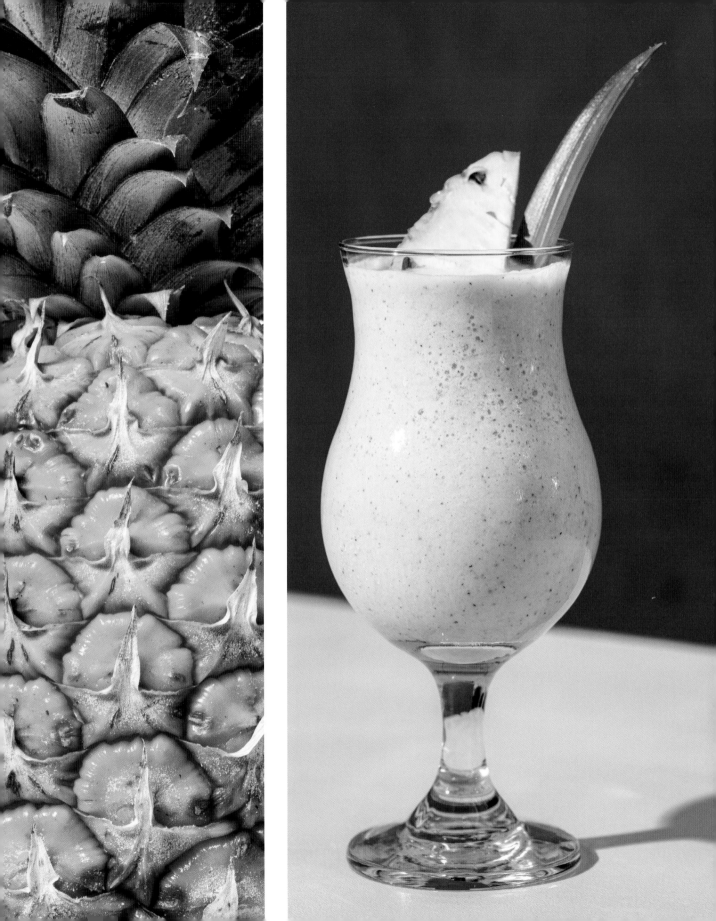

why this combination works: We created an alcohol-free version of the well-loved coconut-based mixed drink, piña colada, with less fat, less sugar, and even a vegetable to boost the nutritional value of this smoothie. Through testing, we found that coconut milk from a can provided the richest coconut flavor when compared against chunks of coconut, coconut water, and coconut milk from a carton. Pineapple chunks proved to be the best way to impart the much-needed pineapple flavor because juice was too liquidy, and the frozen fruit also provided a nice chill. Zucchini had such subtle flavor that it blended in as a neutral background and bulked up the base without masking the tropical flavor. Plus, it left beautiful flecks of green throughout (so there was no need to peel). This smoothie is reminiscent of its inspired cocktail, so you can feel good drinking it, knowing that you're getting fruit, a vegetable, and delicious enjoyment. You won't even miss the rum.

In order listed, add all ingredients to blender and process on low speed until mixture is combined but still coarse in texture, about 10 seconds, scraping down sides of blender jar as needed. Gradually increase speed to high and process until completely smooth, about 1 minute. Adjust consistency with extra water as needed. Serve.

zucchiña colada smoothie

SERVES 2

2 cups frozen pineapple chunks

1 zucchini, chopped coarse

¾ cup water, plus extra as needed

½ cup canned coconut milk

IF YOU DON'T HAVE

frozen pineapple: Use frozen mango chunks or 10 ounces frozen papaya pulp, broken into 1-inch pieces.

zucchini: Use yellow squash.

passionate dragon smoothie

SERVES 2

2½ **cups frozen dragon fruit chunks**

4 **ounces frozen passion fruit pulp, broken into 2-inch pieces**

4 **ounces silken tofu**

½ **ripe banana, peeled**

1 **cup water, plus extra as needed**

why this combination works: Dragon fruit, with its dramatic appearance and exciting name, comes in a variety of internal colors and was a tempting ingredient choice. It had a light, sweet flavor but was ultimately underwhelming. The purply-pink hue from the frozen fruit was too pretty to pass up, though, so we decided to enhance its natural flavor with the assertive taste of tart, tangy passion fruit. The tropical combination was irresistible, with its inviting color and fruity flavor. Blending in banana gave an almost buttery quality to the smoothie that helped balance the tartness of the passion fruit with a mild sweetness. For a creamy emulsifier that disappeared into the drink, we used silken tofu (its plant-based protein was an added boon) and blended everything for a full minute to achieve our desired smooth texture. Passion fruit pulp is often sold in the freezer section with other fruits.

In order listed, add all ingredients to blender and process on low speed until mixture is combined but still coarse in texture, about 10 seconds, scraping down sides of blender jar as needed. Gradually increase speed to high and process until completely smooth, about 1 minute. Adjust consistency with extra water as needed. Serve.

IF YOU DON'T HAVE

frozen passion fruit pulp: Use frozen papaya pulp or frozen mango chunks.

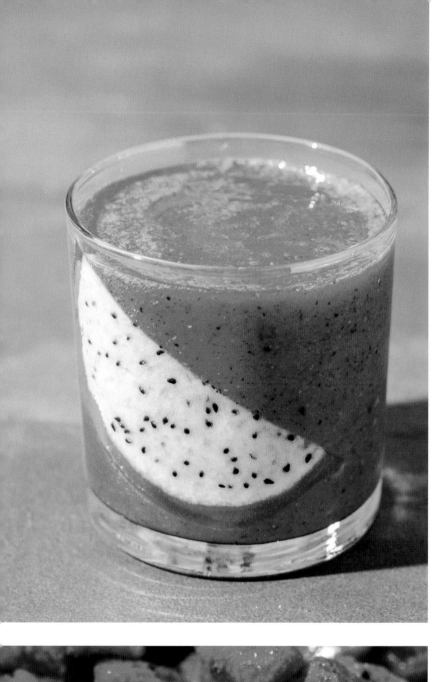
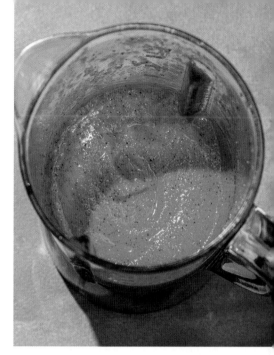
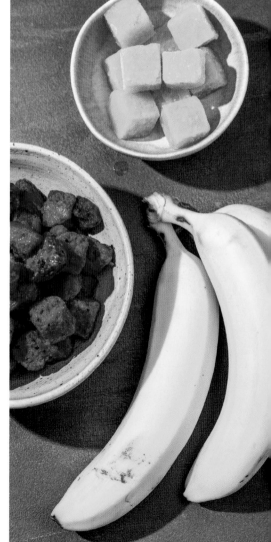
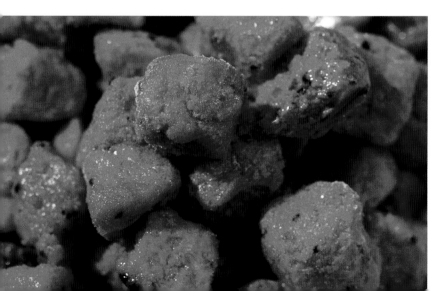

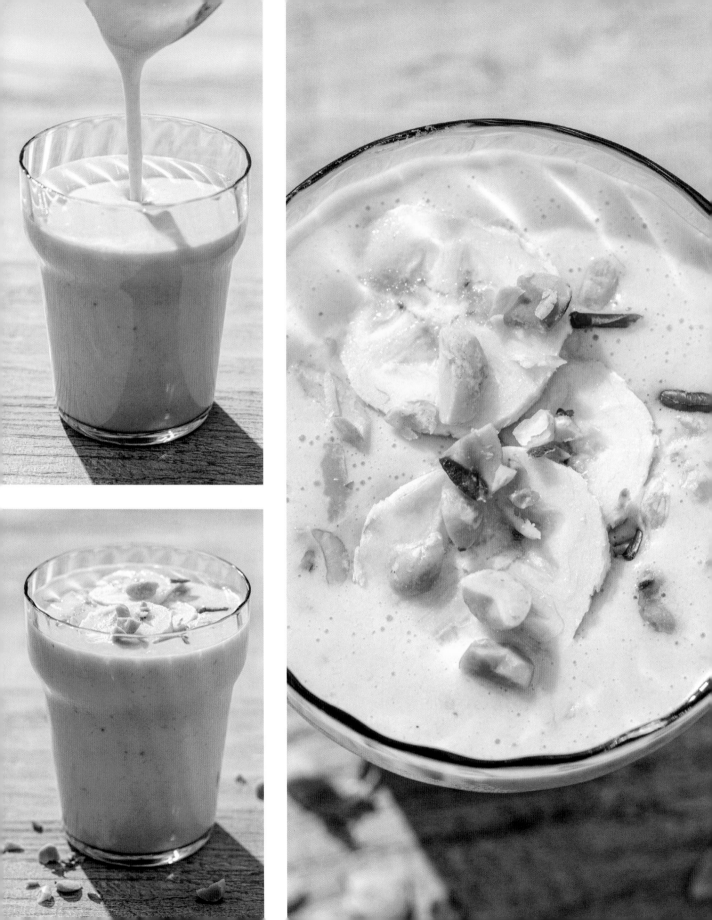

why this combination works: The combination of peanut butter and banana was said to be Elvis's favorite for a reason. The pairing of sweet bananas and salty, creamy peanut butter is an old standby because the flavors contrast so perfectly that they meld into a completely new one, not quite savory and not quite sweet. But because that strong flavor can be easy to overdo, we mellowed the intensity with neutral, creamy yogurt. Bananas, peanut butter, and yogurt all have thick consistencies, so adding a small amount of water was necessary to help the blender blade catch, turn, and process the ingredients properly. We also tested with powdered peanut butter and water and found that it was a perfect swap because the powder had concentrated flavor and the water served as a liquefier. A cooling cup of ice thrown into the blender worked to add aeration and break up the creamy, dense texture. This combination is so good that you could call it the King of Smoothies.

In order listed, add all ingredients to blender and process on low speed until mixture is combined but still coarse in texture, about 10 seconds, scraping down sides of blender jar as needed. Gradually increase speed to high and process until completely smooth, about 1 minute. Adjust consistency with extra water as needed. Serve.

peanut butter-banana smoothie

SERVES 2

1 **cup ice**

2 **ripe bananas, peeled and halved crosswise**

2 **tablespoons creamy peanut butter**

1 **cup plain dairy or plant-based yogurt**

½ **cup water, plus extra as needed**

IF YOU DON'T HAVE

peanut butter: Use other creamy nut or seed butters or powdered peanut butter plus additional water.

ruby red smoothie

SERVES 2

2 tablespoons goji berries

½ cup warm water, plus extra as needed

1 red grapefruit, peeled and quartered

1 cup frozen strawberries

Pinch table salt

½ cup plain dairy or plant-based yogurt

why this combination works: This recipe is loaded with immune-boosting vitamin C and the nutritional powerhouse, goji berries, for a delightfully red, sweet-tart smoothie. Goji berries are a small but mighty fruit that is often overlooked; they resemble cherry tomatoes when fresh and red raisins when dried. Vitamin-rich and antioxidant-loaded, goji berries are most easily found in their dried form, and they taste like a cranberry or sour cherry. For smoother consistency when blending, we rehydrated the goji berries in warm water and then reserved the soaking liquid, full of berry goodness, to use in our smoothie. Combining that tart flavor with sweet frozen strawberries, which made our smoothie cold, and citrusy fresh red grapefruit, which acted like fruit juice but with more fiber, gave us a refreshing, superfood smoothie. We then needed only a pinch of salt and a dollop of yogurt to balance out the drink's bright intensity.

1. Soak goji berries in ½ cup warm water in blender for at least 5 minutes or overnight.

2. Add grapefruit, strawberries, salt, and yogurt to blender (in that order) and process on low speed until mixture is combined but still coarse in texture, about 10 seconds, scraping down sides of blender jar as needed. Gradually increase speed to high and process until completely smooth, about 2 minutes. Adjust consistency with extra water as needed. Serve.

IF YOU DON'T HAVE

goji berries: Use dried cranberries or dried cherries.

strawberries: Use frozen raspberries, blueberries, and/or sweet cherries.

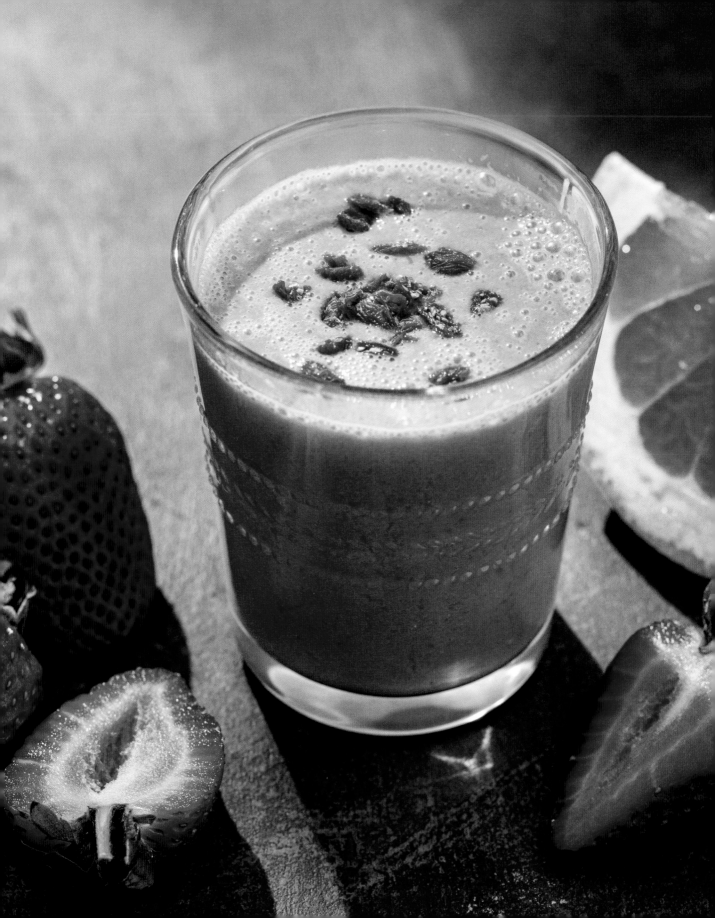

hummingbird smoothie

SERVES 2

- 2 tablespoons raisins
- 1 large carrot, peeled and shredded (¾ cup)
- 1¼ cups frozen pineapple chunks
- 1 tablespoon lucuma powder (optional)
- ¾ cup plain dairy or plant-based yogurt

IF YOU DON'T HAVE

lucuma powder: Omit and increase raisins to ¼ cup.

why this combination works: Taking inspiration from Jamaican hummingbird cake, we sought to echo its tropical, caramelly, and carrot-cake-like flavor in smoothie form. To get this flavor from a shockingly good-for-you source, we employed the antioxidant-rich fruit lucuma, known for its hints of maple and caramel flavors. Famously referred to as the "gold of the Incas," it is readily available in a milder-tasting and shelf-stable powdered form. To draw out its tropical flavors, we combined the lucuma powder with another tropical fruit, pineapple, which we used frozen to keep the smoothie cool and easy to make. After we added shredded carrots and a measured amount of raisins (which we soaked for blendability), the flavor profile began to resemble that of the sweet cake. Yogurt provided creaminess along with a healthy boost of protein for a delicious smoothie that feels more like dessert than a dose of fruits and vegetable.

1. Soak raisins in ½ cup warm water in bowl for at least 5 minutes or overnight; drain.

2. Add raisins, carrot, pineapple, lucuma (if using), yogurt, and 1 cup water to blender (in that order) and process on low speed until mixture is combined but still coarse in texture, about 10 seconds, scraping down sides of blender jar as needed. Gradually increase speed to high and process until completely smooth, about 2 minutes. Adjust consistency with extra water as needed. Serve.

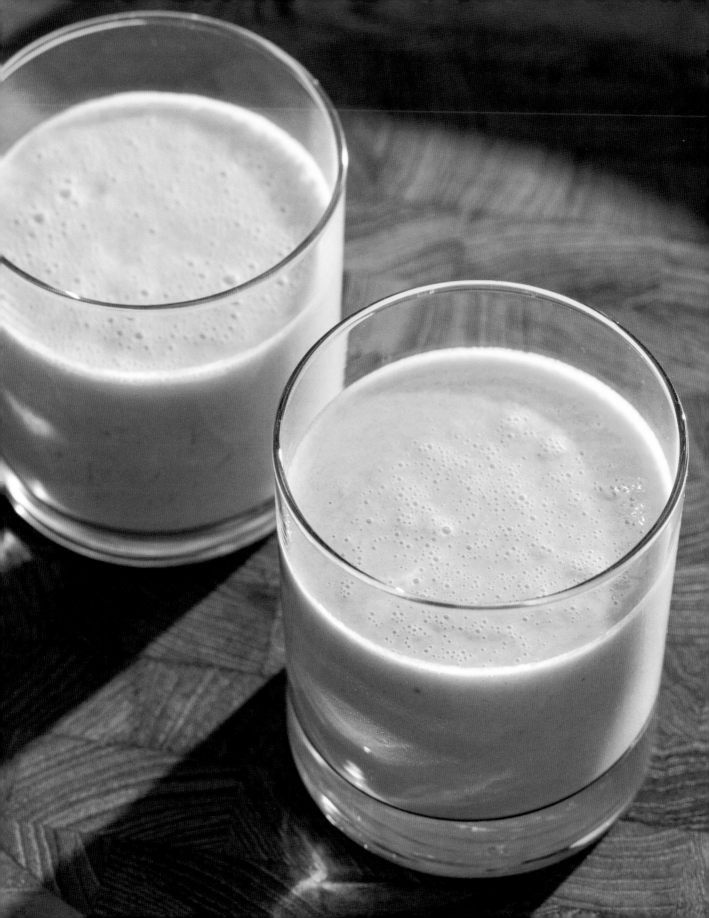

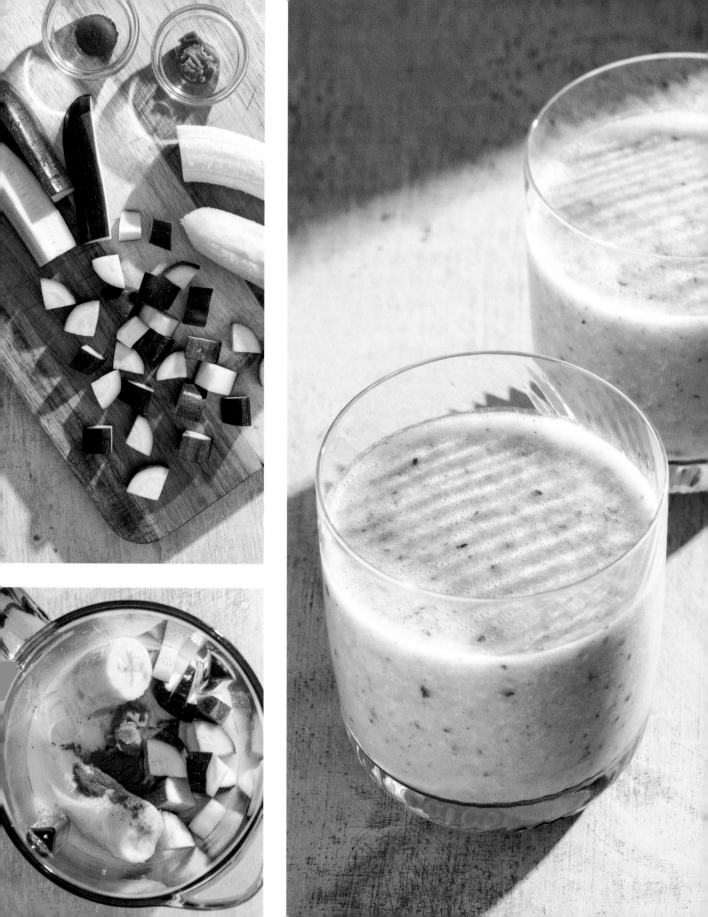

why this combination works: This smoothie is a sweet indulgence with a touch of savory, sophisticated background from miso that makes for an intriguingly delicious drink. We knew that banana was an all-star smoothie ingredient thanks to its versatility, subtle flavor, and desirable texture. Here, it served as a complementary creamy and sweet addition against more vegetal zucchini, which has mild flavor and provides nice bulk. Mixing in milk and a bit of warm spice from cinnamon gave us the added liquid we needed to blend our smoothie and created a baked goods–esque flavor profile (reminiscent of zucchini bread). The unexpected ingredient of salty-tangy miso blended with the banana to elevate our smoothie, giving it a touch of umami and adding a savory nuance to the mild-mannered zucchini.

In order listed, add all ingredients to blender and process on low speed until mixture is combined but still coarse in texture, about 10 seconds, scraping down sides of blender jar as needed. Gradually increase speed to high and process until completely smooth, about 1 minute. Adjust consistency with extra milk as needed. Serve.

miso-banana smoothie

SERVES 2

- 1 **cup ice**

- 1 **medium zucchini, chopped coarse**

- 1 **ripe banana, peeled and halved crosswise**

- 1 **teaspoon white miso**

- ⅛ **teaspoon ground cinnamon**

- 1 **cup dairy or plant-based milk, plus extra as needed**

IF YOU DON'T HAVE

zucchini: Use summer squash.

white miso: Use red miso.

cinnamon: Use pumpkin pie spice blend.

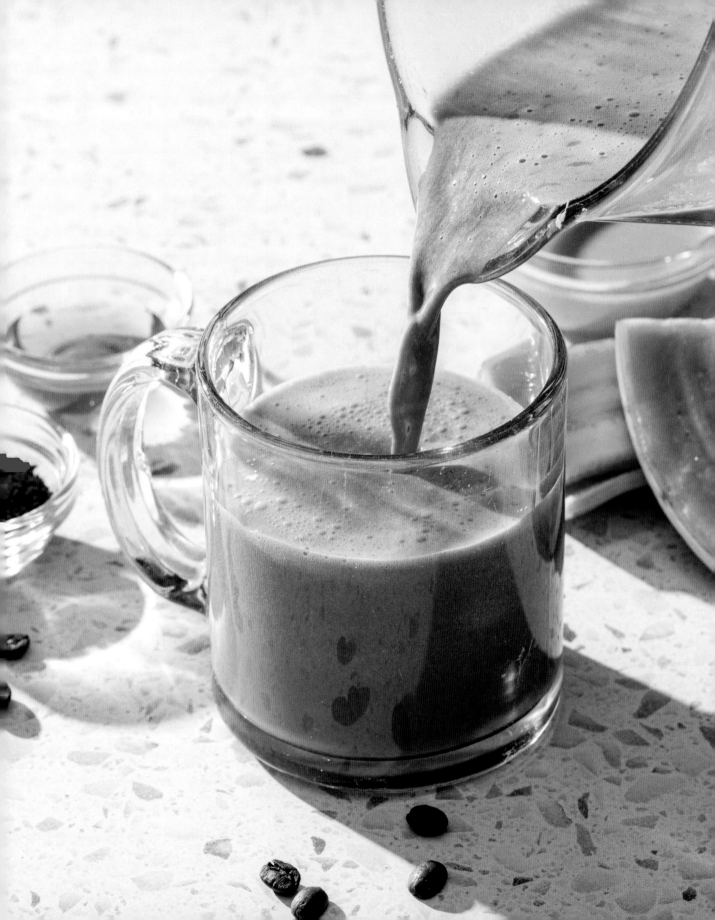

why this combination works: Think of this smoothie like an amped-up Peanut Butter–Banana Smoothie (page 51) but with a honey drizzle—and a strong cup of coffee. Tahini is made from ground sesame seeds and resembles peanut butter but has a looser texture. Like peanut butter, tahini lends nutty smoothness and paired perfectly with body-giving banana as a result. For a sweetener, honey has such concentrated flavor that we needed only 1 tablespoon for its floral-earthy flavor to meld with the tahini. When looking for our coffee element, cold brew and shots of espresso worked, but we loved the ease of instant espresso. Adding a splash of vanilla gave the perception of sweetness without sugar, while a pinch of salt tempered the bitterness of the coffee and enhanced the smoothie's overall flavor. Using half milk and half water as our liquid component rounded out the coffee drink profile by giving it a milkier, richer taste. When blending, 60 seconds was enough to combine the smoothie, but 90 seconds meant that it did not separate while sitting, and it gave us an extra foamy texture, reminiscent of a cappuccino.

In order listed, add all ingredients to blender and process on low speed until mixture is combined but still coarse in texture, about 10 seconds, scraping down sides of blender jar as needed. Gradually increase speed to high and process until completely smooth, about 90 seconds. Adjust consistency with extra milk as needed. Serve.

tahiniccino smoothie

SERVES 2

- 1 **cup ice**
- 1 **ripe banana, peeled and halved crosswise**
- 2 **tablespoons tahini**
- 1 **tablespoon instant espresso powder**
- 1 **tablespoon honey**
- **Pinch table salt**
- 1 **cup dairy or plant-based milk, plus extra as needed**
- 1 **cup water**
- ½ **teaspoon vanilla extract**

IF YOU DON'T HAVE

tahini: Use other creamy seed or nut butters.

instant espresso powder: Use 1 cup cold brew coffee concentrate, cold brew coffee, or cooled strong coffee and omit water.

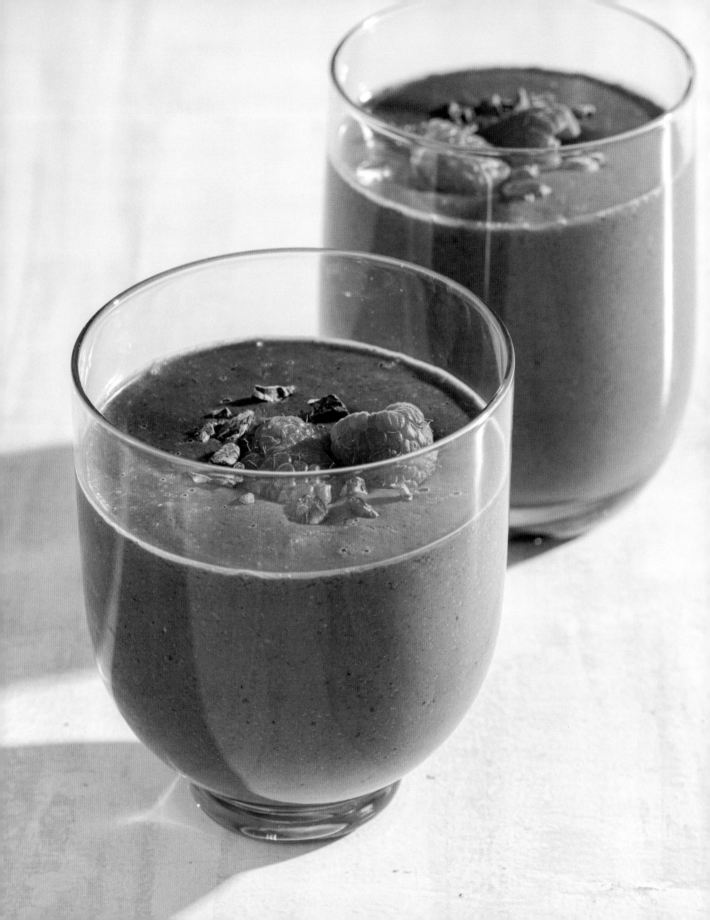

why this combination works: With the classic dessert pairing of chocolate and raspberries in mind, we set out to put them into a drinkable form that indulges your sweet tooth without putting you in a sugar coma. While some tasters didn't like the seeds from the raspberries, we found that they became indistinguishable next to the crunch of cacao nibs. Nicknamed "nature's chocolate chips," cacao nibs are crumbled bits of dried cacao beans, the very same bean used in making chocolate. When it came to our other ingredients, cocoa powder blended chocolaty flavor throughout the smoothie, and banana lived up to its reputation as an all-around hero to add sweet creaminess. Because all these ingredients are a bit dense, we had to add liquid to thin the smoothie but found that water flattened the overall taste. Mixing in almond butter alongside the water provided some depth and toasty roundness that accentuated the chocolate drink flavor. Avoid Dutch-processed cocoa powder as it imparts a bitter taste.

In order listed, add all ingredients to blender and process on low speed until mixture is combined but still coarse in texture, about 10 seconds, scraping down sides of blender jar as needed. Gradually increase speed to high and process until completely smooth, about 2 minutes. Adjust consistency with extra water as needed. Serve.

chocolate-raspberry smoothie

SERVES 2

- 1 cup frozen raspberries
- 1 ripe banana, peeled and halved crosswise
- 2 tablespoons creamy almond butter
- 2 tablespoons cacao nibs
- 2 tablespoons natural unsweetened cocoa powder
- 1½ cups water, plus extra as needed

IF YOU DON'T HAVE

frozen raspberries: Use frozen strawberries, blueberries, blackberries, or sweet cherries.

almond butter: Use other creamy nut or seed butters.

cacao nibs: Omit and increase cocoa powder to 3 tablespoons.

cocoa powder: Omit and increase cacao nibs to ¼ cup.

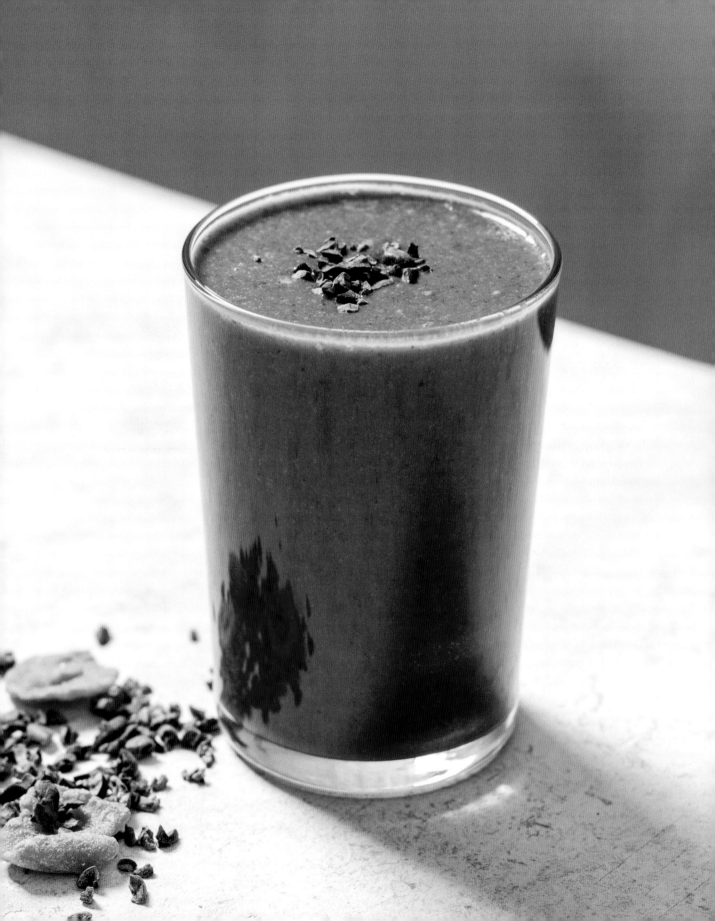

why this combination works: Inspired by red velvet cake, which has vibrant color and a slight cocoa taste, we blended cacao nibs with the ingredient that gives the cake its traditional red color, beets. Cacao nibs are intensely chocolaty but with no added sugar, so when determining whether to pair them with raw or cooked beets, we chose cooked because they were sweeter, and the softer texture let them whip into a smoother consistency. For a more dessert-like base, maple syrup and milk were all we needed to naturally sweeten the smoothie without masking any existing flavors. Our ingredient list brings together all that is Valentine's Day with our last flavor, a splash of rose water. The perfumy, floral taste melted into the rich smoothie to add complexity that is not quite savory and not quite sweet. We had the best success using vacuum-sealed cooked beets; they are typically stored with other prepared fresh produce. Canned beets are also an option; be sure to purchase the unsalted variety and rinse them thoroughly before using. We recommend starting with the lesser amount of rose water and adding more to taste.

In order listed, add all ingredients to blender and process on low speed until mixture is combined but still coarse in texture, about 10 seconds, scraping down sides of blender jar as needed. Gradually increase speed to high and process until completely smooth, about 1 minute. Adjust consistency with extra milk as needed. Serve.

rose velvet smoothie

SERVES 2

- 1 cup ice
- 8 ounces peeled cooked beets, halved
- 3 tablespoons cacao nibs
- 1 tablespoon maple syrup
- 1½ cups dairy or plant-based milk, plus extra as needed
- ¼–½ teaspoon rose water

IF YOU DON'T HAVE

cooked beets: Use peeled and chopped raw beets.

cacao nibs: Use 2 tablespoons natural unsweetened cocoa powder.

maple syrup: Use honey.

cafe mocha smoothie

SERVES 2

2 pitted dates

¼ cup warm water plus ¾ cup cold water

1 cup ice

½ ripe avocado

2 tablespoons cacao nibs

2 tablespoons natural unsweetened cocoa powder

1 tablespoon instant espresso powder

1 cup dairy or plant-based milk, plus extra as needed

IF YOU DON'T HAVE

dates: Omit warm water and substitute 1 ripe banana, peeled and halved crosswise.

cacao nibs: Omit and increase cocoa powder to 3 tablespoons.

cocoa powder: Omit and increase cacao nibs to ¼ cup.

why this combination works: To imitate the coffee-house treat of a caffè mocha, we took the flavors of espresso, milk, and chocolate and combined them with a few creative accompaniments. Espresso and milk were easy enough to come by, so getting the chocolate component just right was the key to this combination. While cacao nibs had the most aromatic flavor and we loved the crunch they gave, the result was not reminiscent of drinking chocolate, so we boosted that chocolatiness with unsweetened cocoa powder. To add creaminess without strong flavor, we used smooth and mild avocado. For a healthful sweetener, dates were the perfect candidate, but they blended up into chunks rather than a smooth paste. Soaking the dates in warm water allowed them to soften and better incorporate when blended for a delectable drink (with some added nutrients). Avoid Dutch-processed cocoa powder as it imparts a bitter taste.

1. Soak dates in warm water in blender for at least 5 minutes or overnight.

2. Add ice, avocado, cacao nibs, cocoa, espresso powder, cold water, and milk to blender (in that order) and process on low speed until mixture is combined but still coarse in texture, about 10 seconds, scraping down sides of blender jar as needed. Gradually increase speed to high and process until smooth, about 90 seconds. Adjust consistency with extra milk as needed. Serve.

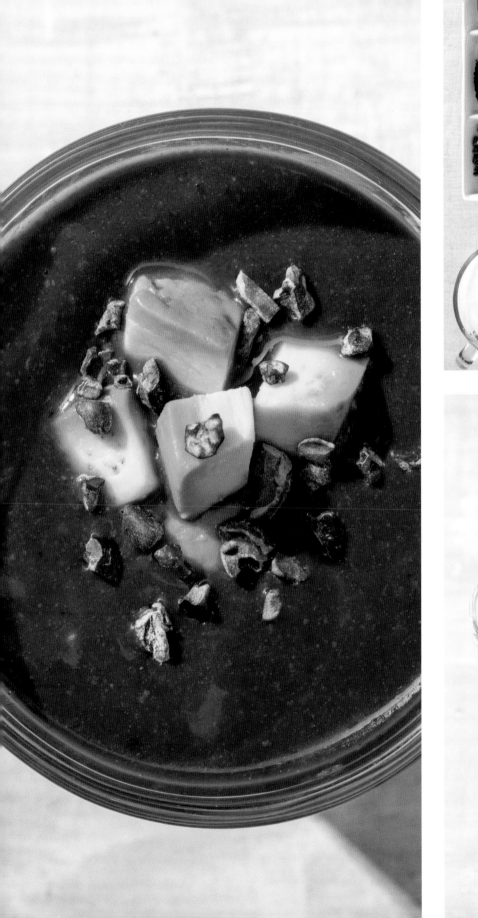

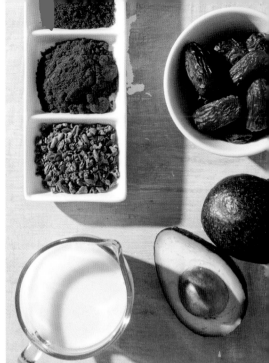

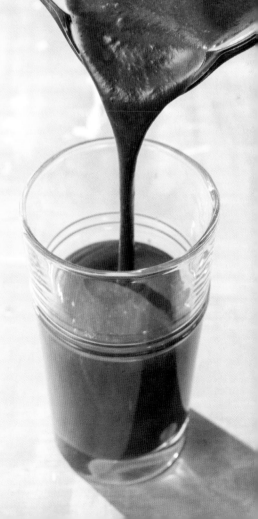

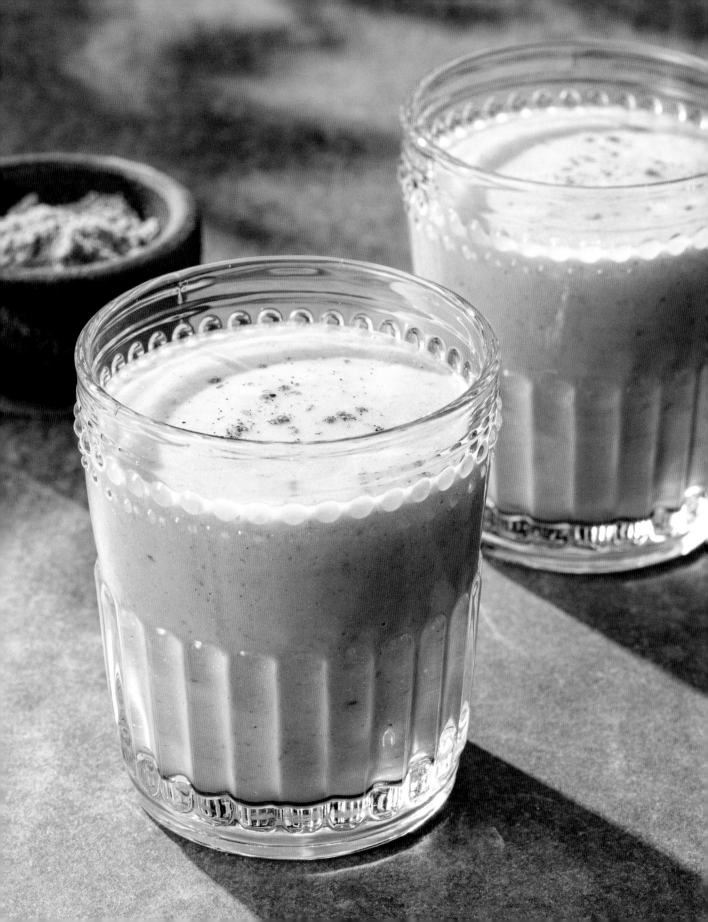

why this combination works: Chestnuts are a distinctive ingredient that don't get enough year-round play, so we looked to create a smoothie that took advantage of their natural properties and holiday spirit. Pairing cooked chestnuts with creamy banana and juicy pear evoked a profile reminiscent of autumnal baked goods that was inviting but left much to be desired in terms of texture. Chestnuts contain very little oil and can be quite fibrous, so they don't break down into a smooth paste. For a more pleasing texture, we added liquid in the form of milk and a few tablespoons of almond butter to make our drink velvety smooth. Ice created some light aeration during blending that turned the thick consistency drinkable. A final touch of ground cardamom solidified our festive flavor for a spirited smoothie that can be drunk during any season. We had the best success using jarred, peeled, cooked chestnuts; they are typically stored with other nuts or dried fruits. They are sometimes referred to as "shelled and ready-to-eat" chestnuts. Do not substitute water chestnuts for the cooked chestnuts.

In order listed, add all ingredients to blender and process on low speed until mixture is combined but still coarse in texture, about 10 seconds, scraping down sides of blender jar as needed. Gradually increase speed to high and process until completely smooth, about 90 seconds. Adjust consistency with extra milk as needed. Serve.

chestnut-pear smoothie

SERVES 2

1 **cup ice**

1 **ripe banana, peeled and halved crosswise**

1 **very ripe pear, peeled, quartered, and cored**

½ **cup peeled cooked chestnuts**

2 **tablespoons creamy almond butter**

¼ **teaspoon ground cardamom**

1¼ **cups dairy or plant-based milk, plus extra as needed**

IF YOU DON'T HAVE

almond butter: Use other creamy nut or seed butters.

cardamom: Use cinnamon.

juices

juicing 101

Juicing is one of the easiest—and most enjoyable—ways to get extra fruits and vegetables into your weekly routine. While supermarkets have a wide variety of ready-to-drink options, they tend to be sugary fruit juices with unnecessary added ingredients. When developing recipes in the test kitchen, we found that the equipment and the quality of the produce greatly impacted the overall experience. There are two kinds of juicers, each with their pros and cons, but both will give you consistently great-tasting homemade juice. Plus, when you juice at home, you can expand your flavor horizons with all the unique tastes and textures that vegetables can bring to your juices. Start your morning with a refreshing glass of Uncommonly Cucumber Juice with Dill (page 82) or try Can't Believe There's Cabbage Juice (page 111) for a drink that is shocking in color and in flavor.

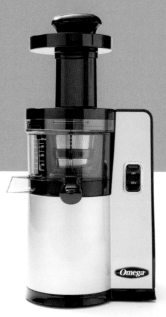

which juicer type is right for you?

CENTRIFUGAL JUICER

- ✓ **Less expensive** (≈$50 to $200)
- ✓ **Faster**
- ✓ **More efficient with dense foods**
- ✓ **Less food prep thanks to wide feed tube**
- ✗ **Loud and messy**
- ✗ **Lower yield from leafy greens**
- ✗ **Juice can be foamy**

MASTICATING JUICER

- ✓ **Quieter**
- ✓ **Less messy**
- ✓ **More efficient with consistently higher yields**
- ✗ **Slower**
- ✗ **More expensive** (≈$300 to $450)
- ✗ **Small feed tube calls for more food prep**

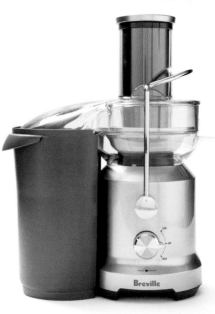

TAKEAWAY

We recommend a centrifugal juicer for people who want to make only a moderate financial investment, and/or don't want to spend time cutting produce down to size. We recommend a masticating juicer for people who are looking for a juicer that is quieter, less messy, and more efficient (especially when dealing with leafy greens).

juicers

WHAT TO USE AND WHAT TO KNOW

All juicers work in roughly the same way: They process fruits and vegetables into pulp and then force the pulp through a fine filtration screen, leaving the solids behind and creating, well, juice. In addition to using our strong winners (the centrifugal **Breville Juice Fountain Cold** and the masticating **Omega VSJ843QS Vertical Low-Speed Juicer**) in the kitchen, we also tested our recipes using a Hamilton Beach centrifugal juicer and an Omega Premium masticating juicer to be sure the juices were replicable with any machine.

WHAT'S THE DIFFERENCE?

The two main types of juicers—centrifugal and masticating—process produce differently. Centrifugal juicers use a shredding disk (like a food processor), which is housed in a finely perforated filter basket. As the food is shredded into pulp, the spinning disk flings the pulp against the sides of the filter basket. The centrifugal force separates the juice, which is dispensed into one container, from the pulp, which is deposited into a second container. Masticating juicers (also called "slow" or "cold-press" juicers) don't have sharp blades. Instead, they use a spinning screw-shaped press called an auger to grind produce into pulp and force it through a fine-mesh filtration screen, squeezing out the juice. Masticating juicers can be horizontal or vertical; the only difference is the placement of their motors and the direction the produce travels in their juicing chambers.

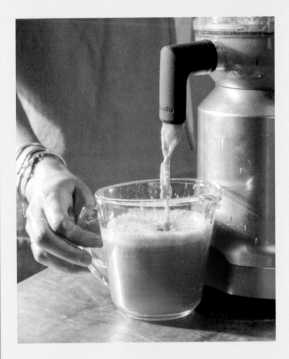

DEBUNKING JUICER MYTHS

As we juiced, we considered two claims people often make about juicers: that centrifugal juicers create warm juice and that the juice produced by masticating juicers stays fresher longer because the machines crush rather than shred produce, preventing oxidation. To see if these claims were true, we measured the internal temperature of carrots before we juiced them and then measured the temperatures of the juices. Centrifugal juicers did not produce notably warmer juice than their masticating counterparts; all temperature changes were within 3 degrees. We also stored 1 cup of carrot juice from each juicer in the refrigerator for four days, photographing and tasting them every day. All the juice samples dulled in flavor and darkened in color over the four days, but *there were no notable differences in taste between juicer types.*

best juicing techniques

fresh is best: For juicing, your produce must be perfectly ripe; as we learned, the older and duller the produce, the lower your yield will be. And too soft isn't great either: You won't get much juice from mushy, overripe fruit. High-quality seasonal produce yields the most juice.

no frozen or hard foods: Frozen fruit will damage the juicer. If you must use frozen fruit, thaw it completely first. Also, a lot of frozen fruit is cut up small. We had better success with bigger slabs of fruits like pineapple. Hard watermelon rind and pineapple rind should be removed before juicing. Remove pits from cherries and other stone fruit.

don't peel! We call for unpeeled produce whenever possible to reduce prep time and increase yield. Sweet potatoes can be peeled if you want a cleaner flavor, but the peel doesn't detract from the overall flavor and doesn't affect the texture of the juice. Clean your produce well before juicing. Think, "Whatever is on it, you are going to drink it."

bundle greens: Pack leafy greens into a tight bundle and fill the feed tube before juicing. You can roll leaves up like a cigar, layering small leaves inside bigger ones. This is especially important for centrifugal juicers.

core pears and apples: It's not because the juicer can't cope but because the seeds have a tiny amount of toxin. You do not want seeds going through the machine.

size matters: Bigger produce ensures a larger yield. Cut as large as possible while still allowing it to fit through the feed tube. Whole tomatoes, cored apples and pears, and big kale leaves will process better than small, chopped pieces.

FOR CENTRIFUGAL JUICERS...

speed matters: Hard produce like beets, sweet potatoes, and carrots need to be juiced on high speed, or they will bounce around. Softer and lighter foods like leafy kale and tomatoes need slow speed, or they'll fly right into the pulp bin. In testing, we doubled our juice yield from tomatoes just by changing to low speed instead of high.

layer ingredients: A basic rule of thumb is heavier and wetter on top of lighter. Add leafy vegetables first, then root vegetables, then pulpy or heavy foods on top, which will weigh things down, so they process better. If you have flavor enhancers, like small pieces of ginger and lemon or extracts, add them earlier so the other produce pushes them through and flushes out as much flavor as possible into your final juice. Otherwise they could get lost.

plunge slowly: In general, slow, steady pushing works best.

FOR MASTICATING JUICERS...

speed does not matter: There is no low or high speed.

adjust your width: Instead of having controllable speed, these juicers have a dial that adjusts the width of the die. The smaller the die, the tighter it squeezes to control the level of extracting.

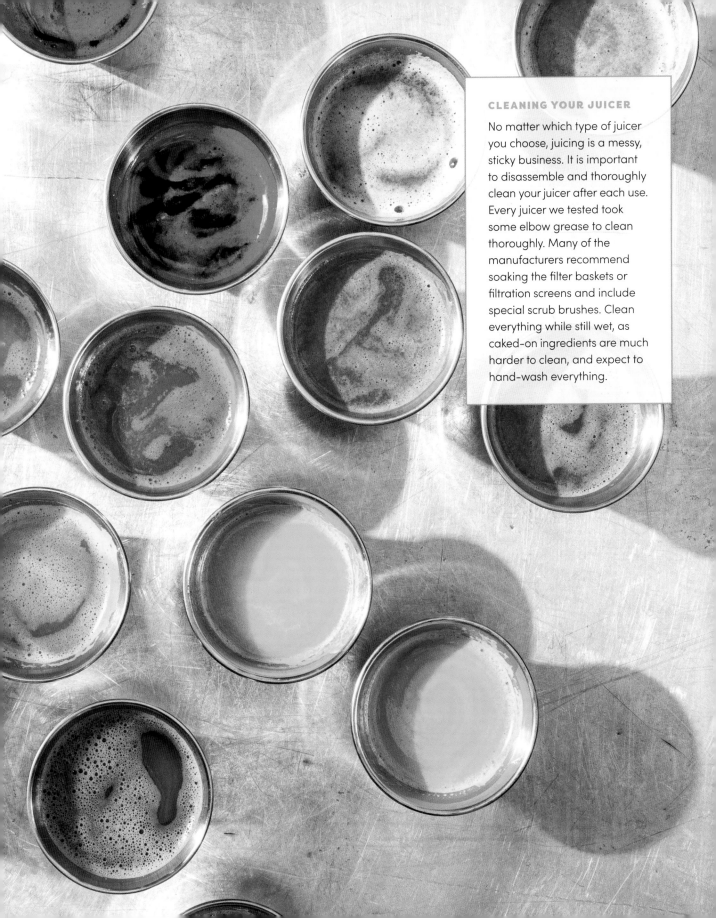

CLEANING YOUR JUICER

No matter which type of juicer you choose, juicing is a messy, sticky business. It is important to disassemble and thoroughly clean your juicer after each use. Every juicer we tested took some elbow grease to clean thoroughly. Many of the manufacturers recommend soaking the filter baskets or filtration screens and include special scrub brushes. Clean everything while still wet, as caked-on ingredients are much harder to clean, and expect to hand-wash everything.

making your own mixes

When you want to branch out from the recipes in this book and experiment with your own combinations, it can be helpful to know the speed at which each type of produce should be juiced. We leave the flavor pairings up to you.

Apples, cored	High
Apricots, pitted	Low
Arugula	High
Beets	High
Berries: *Blueberries, strawberries, and raspberries*	Low
Broccoli	Low
Cabbage	Low
Carrots	High
Celery	High
Cherries, pitted	Low
Cranberries	High
Cucumbers	High
Eggplants	High
Fennel	High
Ginger	High
Grapefruit	Low
Grapes, seedless	Low
Herbs *Parsley, thyme, sage, tarragon, cilantro, mint, and basil*	High
Horseradish root	Low
Jicama	High

Kale	High
Kiwis, peeled	Low
Lemon slice	Low
Lime slice	Low
Mangos, peeled and pitted	Low
Melons, peeled	Low
Nectarines, pitted	Low
Oranges	Low or High
Parsnips	Low
Peaches, pitted	Low
Pears, cored	Low or High
Peppers, bell, seeded	High
Pineapple, peeled	High
Plums, pitted	Low
Romaine lettuce	High
Spinach	High
Sweet potatoes	High
Swiss chard	High
Tomatoes	Low
Turmeric	High
Watercress	High
Watermelon, seedless	Low

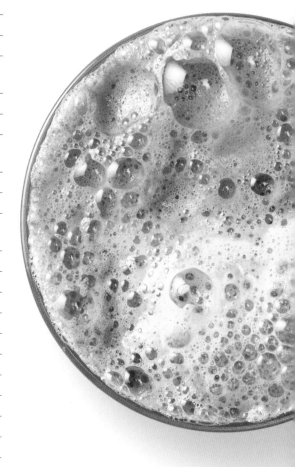

tips for juice making

MIX FLAVORS TO MAKE THEM MORE PALATABLE

Consider pairing sweet veggies or fruit with kale or celery to balance out bitter/vegetal flavors. And if your mixture tastes flat, a spritz of citrus might be just the thing it needs.

USE RESTRAINT

Ginger, turmeric, and horseradish can add a pleasantly spicy note, but don't use too much as the flavor can overwhelm the juice. The same applies to acidic elements like lemon or vinegar: A little goes a long way.

DRIED SPICES OVERPOWER JUICES

Occasionally spices can work in extremely small amounts, but they are frequently too harsh against the delicate flavors of the juice. If you try them, start with the smallest amount possible and work your way up.

YOU DRINK WITH YOUR EYES FIRST

Think about layering colors to make a pretty ombre drink, or incorporating a brightly colored ingredient for a vibrant juice.

STORAGE AND SHELF LIFE OF JUICE

Some people like making and storing larger batches of juice, but based on how the flavors of our samples changed, we don't recommend storing juice for longer than 24 hours, regardless of which style of juicer you use. Within 12 hours, the juice may lose its vibrancy and start to dull in color and flavor. Within as little as 30 minutes the juice sediment will start to settle, so whisk vigorously before drinking.

TEST KITCHEN DISCOVERY

get the most out of your citrus

While working on this chapter, we discovered the perfect way to infuse our drinks with citrus flavor. Cut citrus fruits into ¼-inch rounds and use a centrifugal juicer on low speed so the teeth can perfectly zest the outside and juice the inside. The pith is spit out largely intact, so there is no bitter, acrid taste. You extract everything you want and leave what you don't. The size of the slice really matters: Too thin and it flies out into the waste tube; too thick and you crush too much of the pith. Citrus slices work in a masticating juicer too, but it does not zest the fruit at all. You have to quarter grapefruit slices in order to fit.

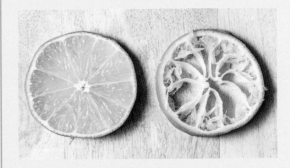

WE FAILED SO YOU DON'T HAVE TO

We tried juicing certain ingredients that had some very unpleasant results. Bananas and persimmons produced an unpleasant, thick texture. Mangos and papayas gave very low yield and lacked a good, concentrated flavor. Eggplants turned out bitter with a murky color, while alliums like garlic and chives overwhelmed all other flavors.

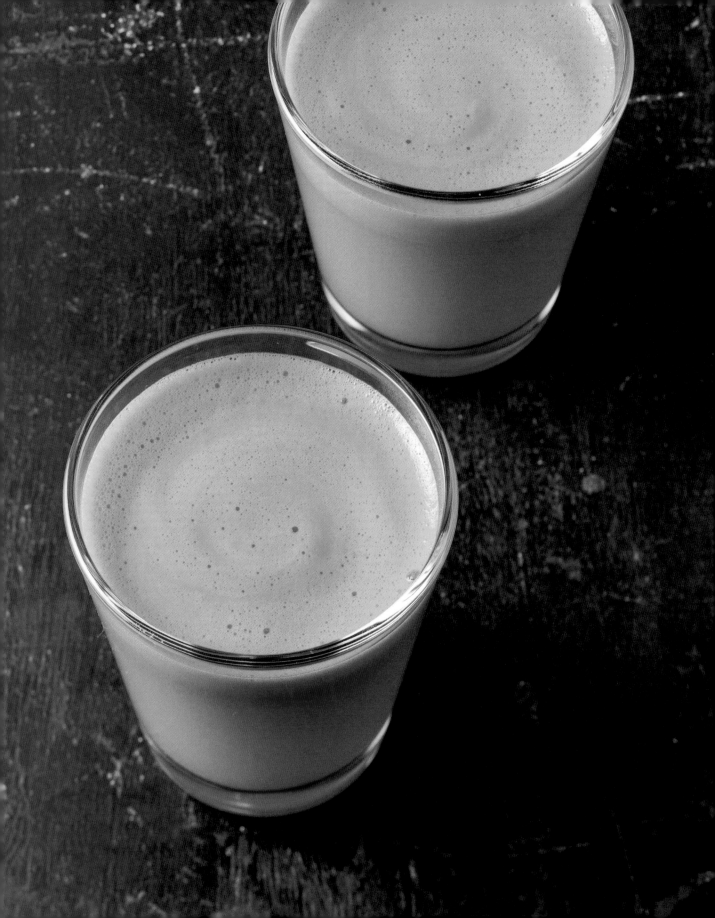

why this combination works: While we can't promise that this drink will improve your eyesight, we love juiced carrots because they taste both sweet and savory. The process of juicing creates an ultraconcentrated carrot flavor that you can enjoy all on its own, or take in a multitude of directions. We found peeled versus unpeeled carrots had little to no flavor difference, so we left them unpeeled to cut down on prep time. Some of our variations included citrus, and we discovered a great new trick: Put a sliced round of citrus fruit in a juicer on low speed and the machine zests the rind, juices the fruit, and spits out the pith, adding delicious flavor without any bitterness. For a punchy variation, we added a slice of lemon and a bit of ginger to the carrot. For a version with complementary acidic tones and enhanced fruitiness, we juiced grapefruit and carrot together. And for a totally no-prep juice, we threw in the carrot greens along with the roots. Juicing the carrots with their greens still intact paired perfectly with a touch of balsamic vinegar for a fresh taste reminiscent of a summery salad.

On high speed, process carrots through juicer into storage container or serving glass. Serve.

VARIATIONS

with lemon and ginger
On low speed, process 1 (¼-inch-thick) slice lemon. Increase speed to high and process 1 (1-inch) piece ginger and carrots. Stir to combine before serving.

with grapefruit
Reduce carrots to 1 pound. On low speed, process 1 (¼-inch-thick) slice grapefruit, halved. Increase speed to high and process carrots. Stir to combine before serving.

with carrot greens and balsamic
On high speed, process 1 cup carrot greens and carrots (in that order) . Stir in ¾ teaspoon balsamic vinegar before serving.

completely carrot juice

SERVES 1 TO 2

1¼   **pounds carrots, unpeeled**

IF YOU DON'T HAVE

carrot greens: Use 2 ounces baby arugula.

balsamic vinegar: Use white wine vinegar or apple cider vinegar.

feel the
beet juice

SERVES 1 TO 2

**1 pound beets, unpeeled,
trimmed**

why this combination works: Knowing beets to be the superfood they are, we set out to develop recipes that made them both easy and enticing to drink. Beets have a slew of health benefits, and we loved the straightforward flavor of unaltered juiced beets. Rather than disguising the taste of beets, we leaned into their distinctly earthy-sweet notes by juicing them unpeeled (plus: less prep). Though we found the plain beet juice quite drinkable, we knew that their unique taste doesn't appeal to everyone, so we created a few flavorful variations. First, we tested warm spices and found that allspice, with its nutty versatility, worked best with the beets, and adding orange juice to the mix yielded a juice that tasted almost like Angostura bitters. Our second blend combined juicy sweet grapes with fresh thyme's subtle herbal notes. For a third juice that utilized both the beet root and greens, we turned to pear, which added nice body, flavor, and sweetness to balance the bitterness of the beet greens.

On high speed, process beets through juicer into storage container or serving glass. Serve.

VARIATIONS
with orange and allspice
On low speed, process 1 (¼-inch-thick) slice orange. Increase speed to high and process beets. Stir in pinch ground allspice before serving.

with grapes and thyme
On low speed, process ½ cup seedless grapes and 5 sprigs fresh thyme. Increase speed to high and process beets. Stir to combine before serving.

with beet greens and pear
Reduce beets to 12 ounces. On high speed, process ½ cored pear, 4 ounces beet greens, and beets (in that order). Stir to combine before serving.

IF YOU DON'T HAVE

beet greens: Use Swiss chard leaves and stems.

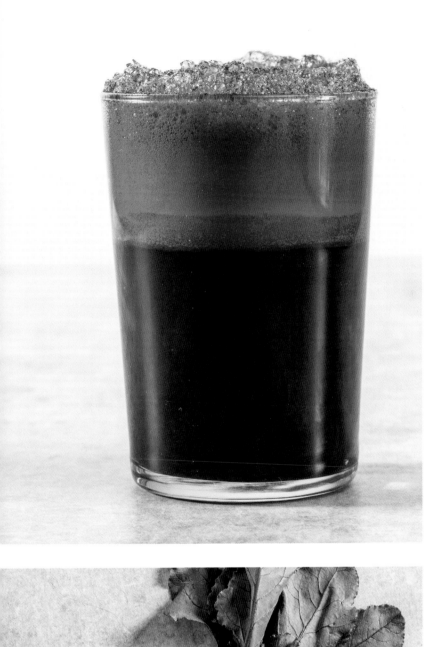
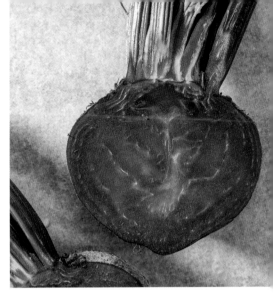
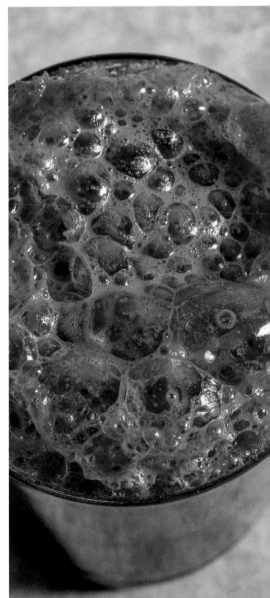
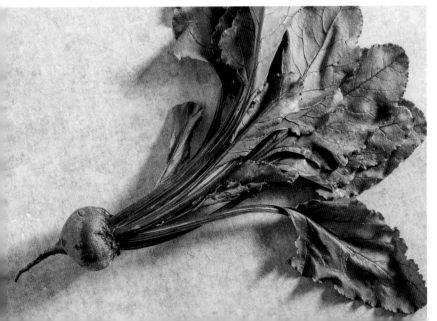

seriously celery juice

SERVES 1 TO 2

12 ounces celery

why this combination works: Celery as an ingredient often seems to play second fiddle, with its main attributes being crunchy, stringy, and mildly savory, but juicing it was a revelation. Fresh celery juice has a clean sweetness and salinity that tastes and feels like it's good for you. By itself, it turns a surprisingly deep green and is immensely appealing when you're looking for healthful hydration in the form of a morning pick-me-up. We found that celery plays very well with fruits, and that it was particularly pleasing when paired with acidic partners and herbal additions. We first mixed in zippy lemon juice and licoricey fennel, and then green apple and tarragon to produce a juice with a slightly sweeter profile. Our final variation added syrupy strawberries for nuanced sweet, salty, and berryish notes.

On high speed, process celery through juicer into storage container or serving glass. Serve.

VARIATIONS
with fennel and lemon
Reduce celery to 8 ounces. On low speed, process 1 (¼-inch-thick) slice lemon. Increase speed to high and process ½ small fennel bulb and celery (in that order). Stir to combine before serving.

with green apple and tarragon
Reduce celery to 8 ounces. On high speed, process ¼ cup fresh tarragon and tender stems, ½ cored green apple, and celery (in that order). Stir to combine before serving.

with strawberry
Reduce celery to 9 ounces. On low speed, process 5 ounces hulled strawberries. Increase speed to high and process celery. Stir to combine before serving.

IF YOU DON'T HAVE

lemon: Use lime.

tarragon: Use parsley or basil.

green apple: Use any apple or pear.

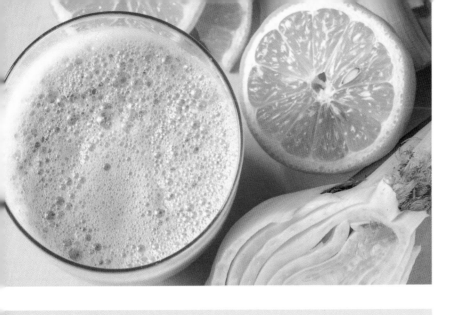

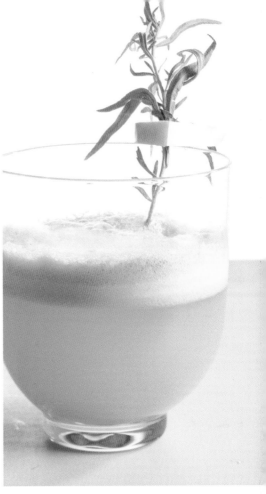

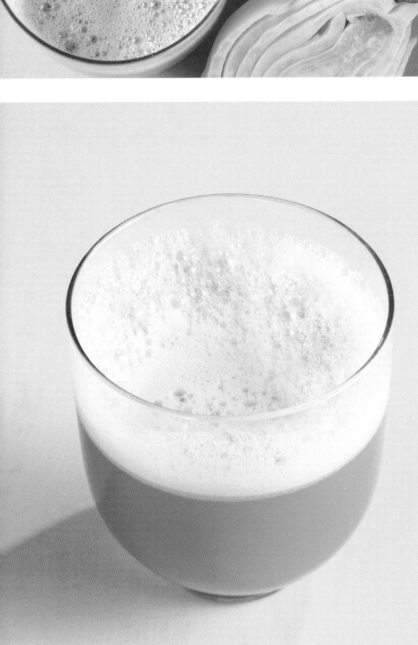

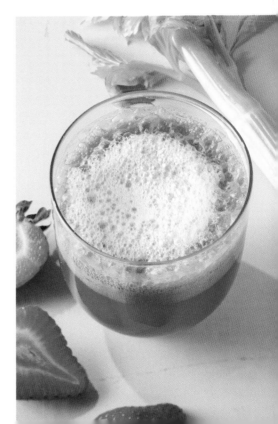

uncommonly cucumber juice

SERVES 1 TO 2

12 ounces cucumbers, unpeeled

why this combination works: Cucumber's clean, refreshing taste translates into a bracing veggie juice. When juicing cucumbers, we used big unpeeled pieces and cut them only if needed to fit through the juicer because the larger size gave the machine something to grab on to. We kept the skins on because they contributed vibrant color and fuller flavor, not to mention making prep easier. In lieu of peeling, we took good care to scrub them, because cucumbers can have a waxy coating to protect them from deteriorating. While cucumber juice is a perfectly pure expression of the vegetable, it also makes an adaptable base to choose your own adventure. Mint and lime reminded us of a mojito (hold the hangover). Sea salt and chile evoked a smashed Chinese cucumber salad. And cucumber juice with the simple addition of dill made us happily think of dill pickles. Any variety of cucumber will work in this recipe.

On high speed, process cucumbers through juicer into storage container or serving glass. Serve.

VARIATIONS
with mint and lime
On low speed, process 1 (¼-inch-thick) slice lime and ¾ cup fresh mint and tender stems. Increase speed to high and process cucumber. Stir to combine before serving.

with sea salt and chile
On high speed, process 1 stemmed and seeded Thai chile and cucumber (in that order). Stir pinch sea salt into juice before serving.

with dill
On high speed, process ½ cup fresh dill and tender stems and cucumber (in that order).

IF YOU DON'T HAVE

lime: Use lemon.

Thai chile: Use ½ seeded jalapeño or Fresno chile.

dill: Use tarragon.

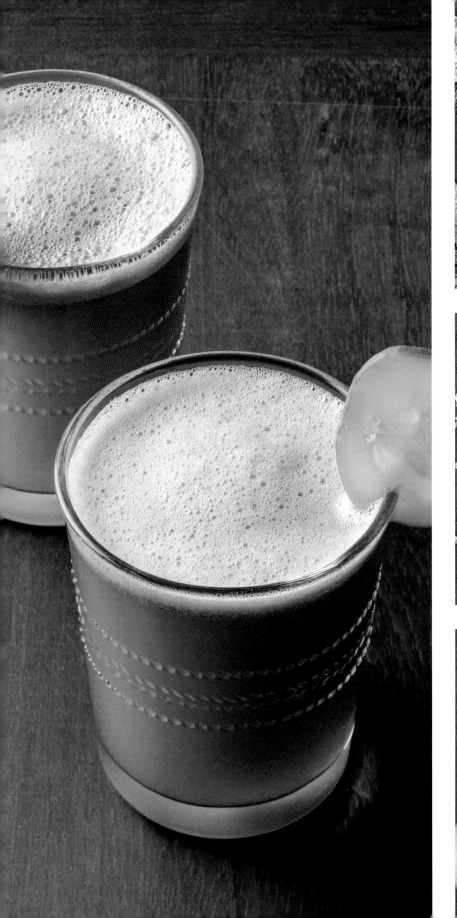
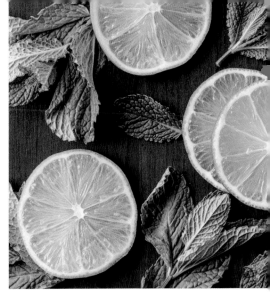
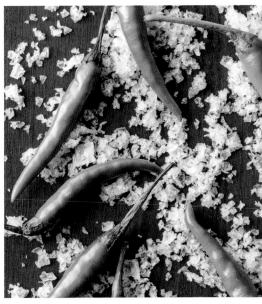
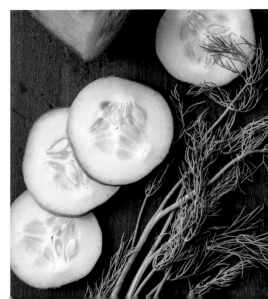

totally tomato juice

SERVES 1 TO 2

1 pound tomatoes

IF YOU DON'T HAVE

fresh herbs: Use cilantro for parsley. Use tarragon for basil.

fresh horseradish: Use 1 teaspoon prepared horseradish.

peach: Use 1 nectarine.

why this combination works: A beloved favorite of airplane travelers and boozy brunches, tomato-based drinks are deliciously savory anywhere, anytime. Although juicing typically filters out the bulk of most solids, tomatoes are so tender that much of their flesh passes through the juicer to produce a silky, thicker juice. Fresh tomato juice, without the additives found in store-bought versions, is so appetizingly salty and clean-tasting that you'll find yourself finishing a glass and immediately going back for another. To play up the tomato's piquant quality, we made one variation with bright lemon and a big handful of parsley that tastes delightfully herbaceous. Giving a nod to its brunchy Bloody Mary connection, tomato juice also blended perfectly with the flavors of fresh horseradish and freshly ground black pepper. For a sweeter take, our last variation used peach to bring out the fruity quality of tomatoes while still adding a faintly savory finish with some fresh basil. Any variety of tomato will work in this recipe.

On low speed, process tomatoes through juicer into storage container or serving glass. Serve.

VARIATIONS
with lemon and parsley
On low speed, process 1 (¼-inch-thick) slice lemon, 1 cup fresh parsley and tender stems, and tomatoes (in that order). Stir to combine before serving.

with horseradish and black pepper
On low speed, process 1 (¼-inch) piece fresh horseradish root and tomatoes (in that order). Stir ½ teaspoon pepper into juice before serving.

with peach and basil
Reduce tomatoes to 12 ounces. On low speed, process 1 peach, halved and pitted, ½ cup fresh basil and tender stems, and tomatoes (in that order). Stir to combine before serving.

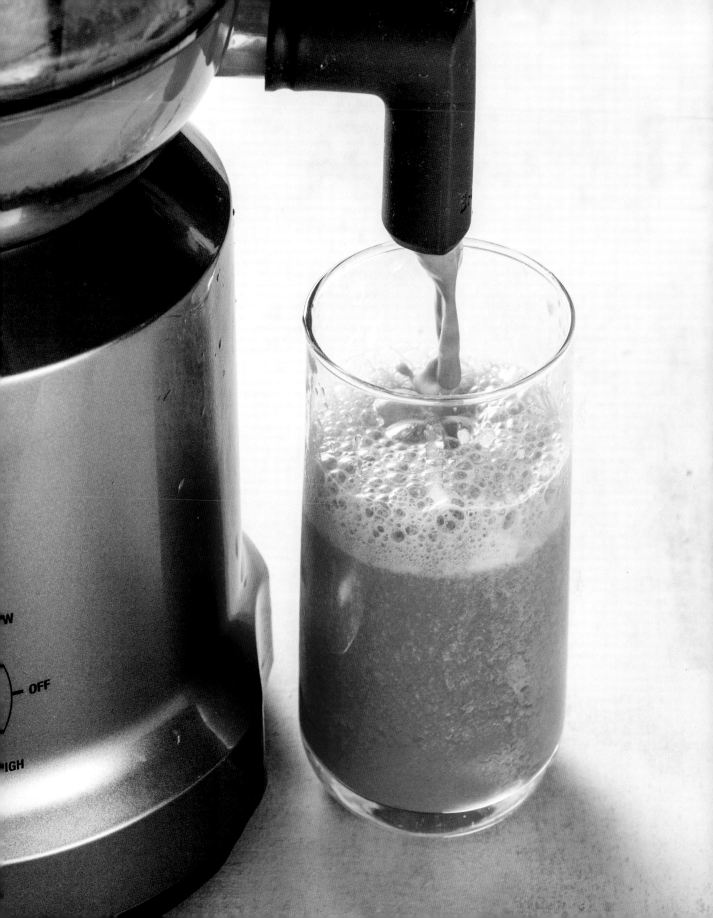

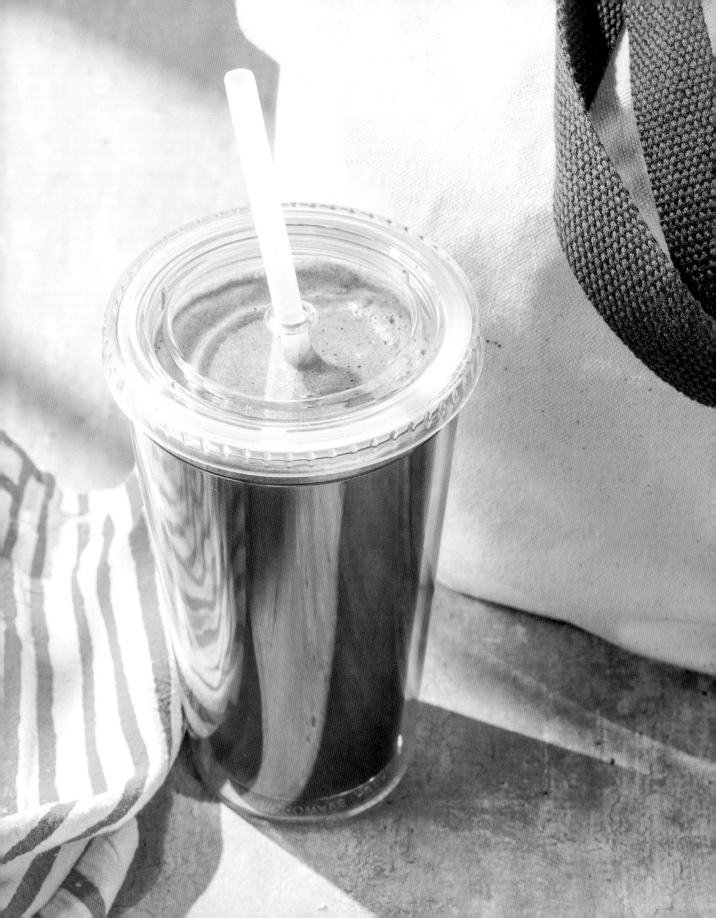

why this combination works: When done right, juices filled with nutrient-rich green produce can be a flavorful way to get extra vitamins and minerals into your daily diet. This introductory green juice doesn't skimp on vegetal content but has a well-balanced, drinkable flavor that you'll want to reach for. Parsley and lacinato kale, also known as Tuscan kale, served as the base for our juice, with parsley bringing a grassy brightness to balance the more bitter kale. Celery added savory volume to the drink thanks to its high water content and also helped subdue the intense kale flavor. Our fourth green ingredient came in the form of a green apple, which contributed a sweet-tart tang to mellow the greens. Lemon and ginger, a common pairing in juices, worked to enhance the greens by adding some acidity and lively spicy notes. For more information on processing hearty leafy greens, see page 72.

On low speed, process lemon through juicer into storage container or serving glass. Increase speed to high. In order listed, process remaining ingredients. Stir to combine before serving.

daily greens juice

SERVES 1 TO 2

1 (¼-inch-thick) slice lemon

1 (½-inch) piece fresh ginger

½ cup fresh parsley and tender stems

4 ounces lacinato kale

½ green apple, cored

2 celery ribs

IF YOU DON'T HAVE

lemon: Use lime.

parsley: Use cilantro.

lacinato kale: Use 8 ounces curly kale.

green apple: Use any apple.

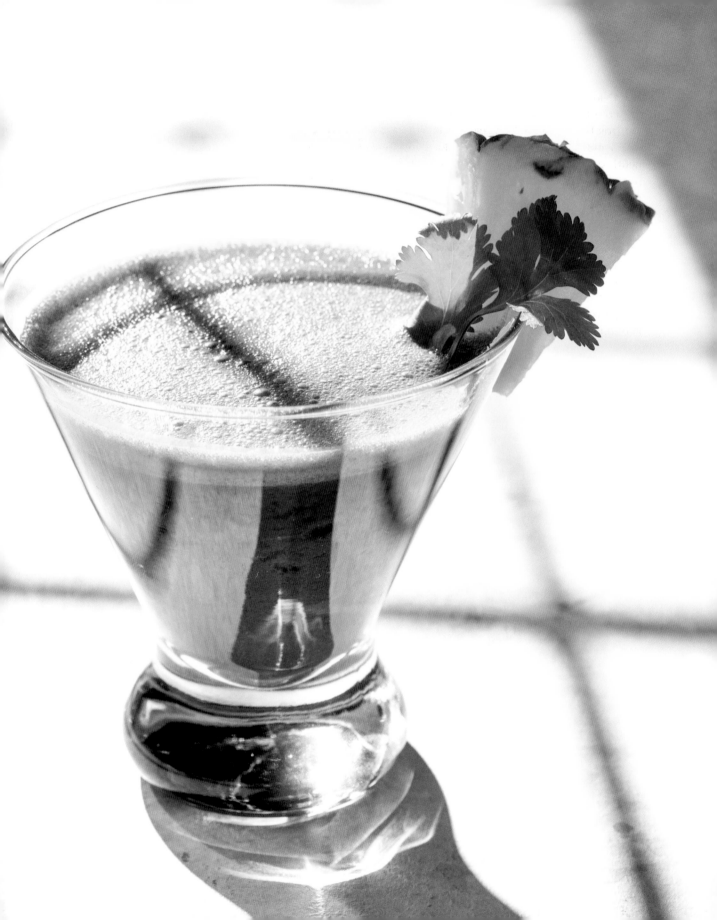

why this combination works: During our smoothie endeavors, we discovered our love for pineapple in drinks because of its immediately recognizable tropical, acidic flavor, so we created a juice that utilizes it as a complementary ingredient alongside a hearty green. While kale can be accused of tasting aggressively healthy, it needs only a few other ingredients to work as a great green backdrop to bolder flavors. Pineapple is a naturally juicy fruit, so when put through a juicer, much of its body made its way through the machine to become a thickened juice that held on to the kale flavor while subduing its intensity. The addition of a yellow bell pepper and cilantro gave the pineapple and kale another kick of sweetness as well as an herbal component that complemented the fruit, as it would in a mixed drink, without being overly cilantro-esque (even for cilantro haters). For more information on processing hearty leafy greens, see page 72.

On high speed and in order listed, process ingredients through juicer into storage container or serving glass. Stir to combine before serving.

pineapple-kale juice

SERVES 1 TO 2

4 **ounces lacinato kale**

½ **cup fresh cilantro and tender stems**

1 **yellow bell pepper, halved, stemmed, and seeded**

4 **ounces peeled pineapple**

IF YOU DON'T HAVE

lacinato kale: Use 8 ounces curly kale.

cilantro: Use parsley.

yellow bell pepper: Use any color bell pepper.

cucumber and kiwi juice

SERVES 1 TO 2

1 kiwi, peeled

¾ cup fresh mint leaves and tender stems

5 ounces curly-leaf spinach

5 ounces cucumber, unpeeled

why this combination works: While green juices can be dense with vegetal bulk, this lighter and brighter take relies on cucumber, kiwi, and spinach as our green produce. Cucumber and kiwi are similarly aromatic, with one savory and the other sweet. Their complementary flavors combined to create an entirely new one that landed somewhere in the middle. Plus, they produced a lot of liquid to create a light, refreshing mixture. Fragrant fresh mint added a coolness and tied the flavors together, while mildly grassy spinach contributed depth, nutrition, and some subtly appealing bitterness. For more information on processing hearty leafy greens, see page 72. Any variety of cucumber will work in this recipe.

On low speed, process kiwi through juicer into storage container or serving glass. Increase speed to high. In order listed, process remaining ingredients. Stir to combine before serving.

IF YOU DON'T HAVE

curly-leaf spinach: Use baby spinach.

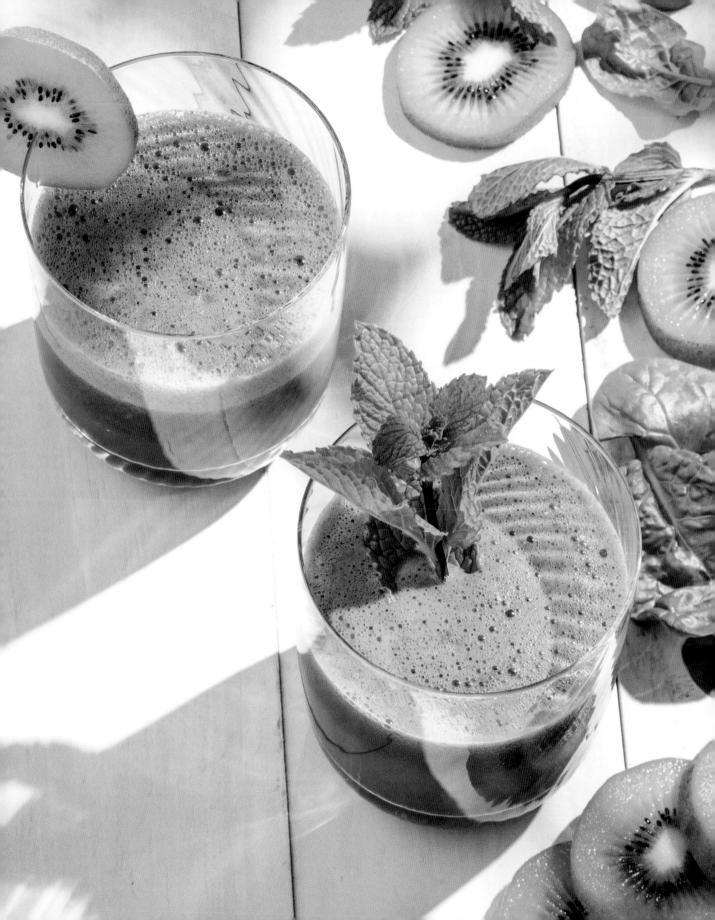

sweet corn and blueberry juice

SERVES 2

¾ cup (1 ear) fresh corn kernels

1 cup blueberries

5 ounces Swiss chard

IF YOU DON'T HAVE

fresh corn: Use thawed frozen corn.

blueberries: Use blackberries, raspberries, or strawberries.

Swiss chard: Use curly-leaf spinach or baby spinach.

why this combination works: This juice invokes the fresh flavors that come from peak-of-summer produce. Corn juice (a term you may not have heard before) is amazingly sweet and surprisingly starchy, so it provided a thickening quality that gave this juice combo an almost smoothie-like texture. To make the flavor profile more complex while adding welcome tartness, antioxidant-rich blueberries did just the trick and also turned our juice a beautiful purply shade. We loved this pairing but found it still a little too sweet, so we knew we had to add an ingredient that would offset the concentrated flavor without detracting from it. The slight bitterness of dark, leafy Swiss chard melted into the background and gave the drink a hint of vegetal flavor that made the juice more appealing. For more information on processing hearty leafy greens, see page 72.

On low speed, process corn and blueberries through juicer into storage container or serving glass. Increase speed to high and process chard. Stir to combine before serving.

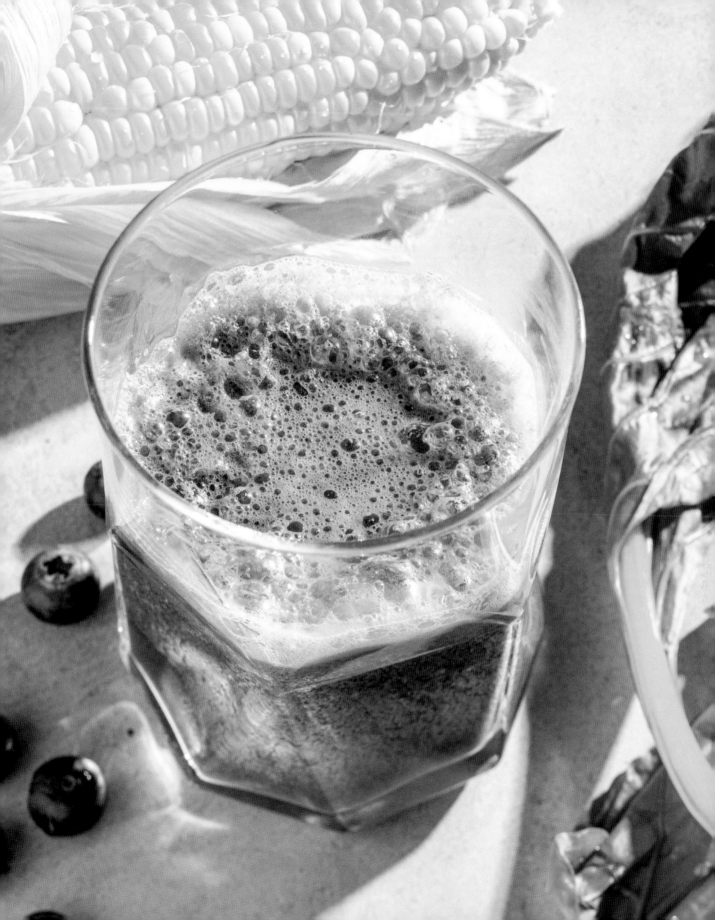

spicy jicama juice with lime

SERVES 1 TO 2

2 (¼-inch-thick) slices lime

5 ounces curly-leaf spinach

½ Fresno chile, seeded

14 ounces jicama, peeled

Coarse sea salt

why this combination works: Uniquely piquant, this juice was inspired by the popular Mexican snack of spicy jicama sticks with lime juice and tajín (or chili powder). Jicama, which is high in water content, supplied our juice with a sweet and starchy backbone. We knew we wanted to incorporate a green, but because jicama's sweetness is subtle, we didn't want to overwhelm it. Spinach turned out to be our just-right Goldilocks green, combining nicely with the jicama and adding vegetal flavor without much bitterness. For our spicy kick, we eschewed dry spices like tajín or cayenne because the flavor felt muted in the juice, whereas a fresh Fresno chile added an ideal level of spicy clarity. The lime juice worked to brighten the vegetables and balance the heat from the chile, while flaky sea salt gave us a well-rounded and stimulating drink.

On low speed, process lime through juicer into storage container or serving glass. Increase speed to high and process spinach, chile, and jicama (in that order). Stir to combine and sprinkle with salt before serving.

IF YOU DON'T HAVE

curly-leaf spinach: Use baby spinach.

Fresno chile: Use jalapeño chile.

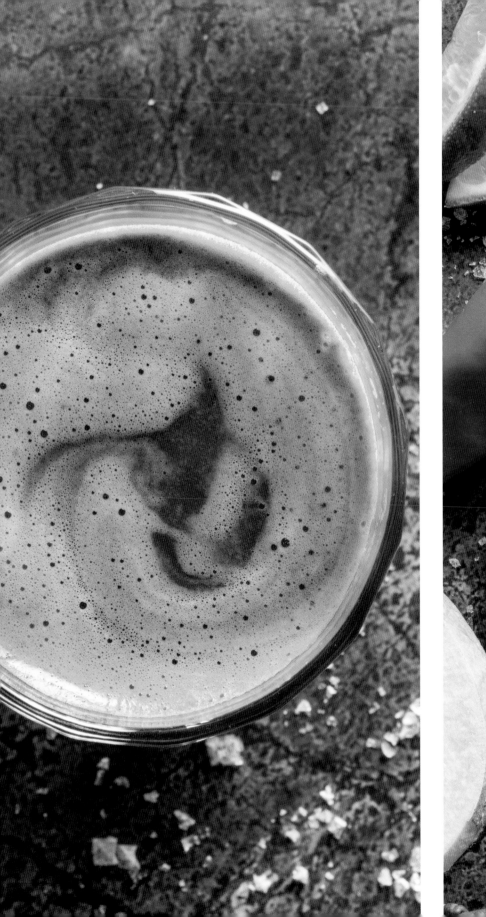
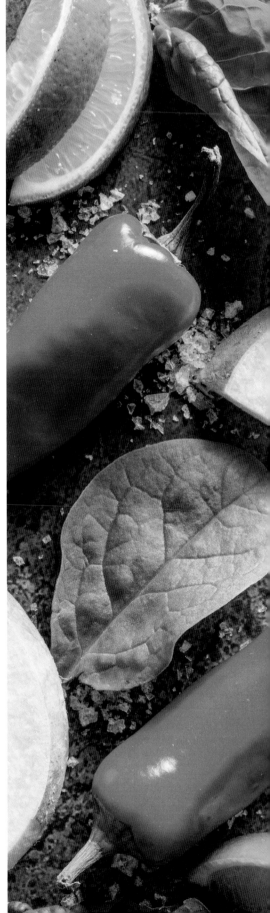

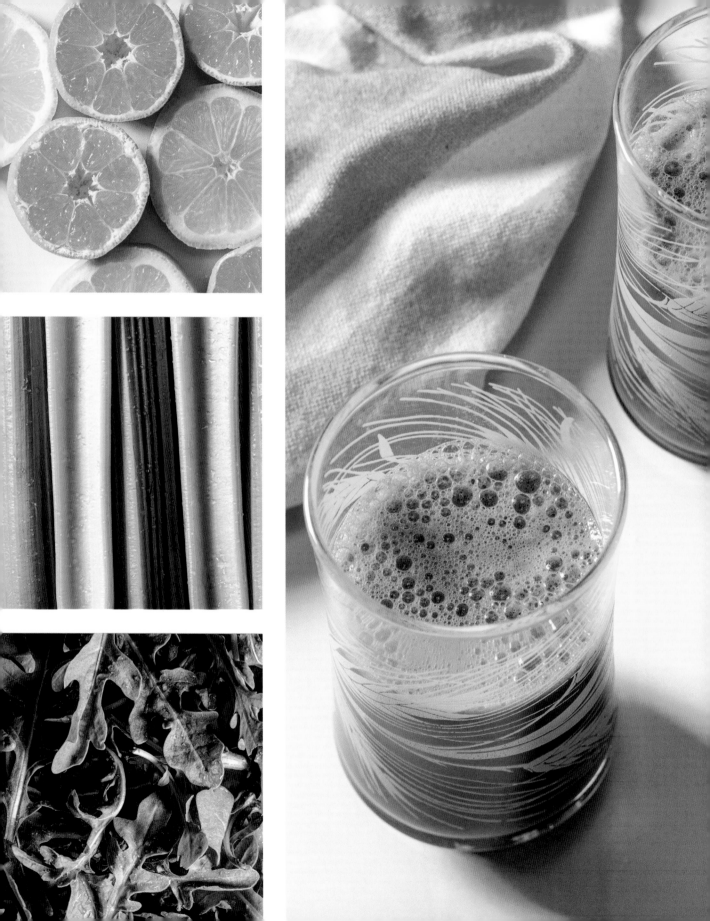

why this combination works: This invigorating juice is ideal to serve at your next brunch gathering or to enjoy solo to jump-start your morning with a peppery kick. Though you might expect this juice to be sour, the dominant flavor comes from spicy arugula. Baby arugula has a particularly mustardy punch that hits the mouth and travels up through the nose to awaken your taste buds and senses. We loved this quality but wanted to tamp it down slightly to make it more drinkable. Juiced celery ribs gave our juice a grassy and savory backbone that relaxed the arugula taste but still kept the flavor distinctly green. To tone down the sting of vegetal pepperiness but still keep the greenness front and center, we tested different citrus fruits that would brighten and gently sweeten the drink. Mandarin oranges are sweeter than standard oranges and therefore mix delightfully with fresh lemon juice for a complex and punchy citrus flavor without a sour shock.

On low speed, process lemon through juicer into storage container or serving glass. Increase speed to high. In order listed, process remaining ingredients. Stir to combine before serving.

citrus burst and arugula juice

SERVES 1 TO 2

1 (¼-inch-thick) slice lemon

3 ounces baby arugula

2 mandarin oranges, peeled

4 celery ribs

IF YOU DON'T HAVE

mandarin oranges: Use 2 tangelos, 1 navel orange, or 3 clementines.

atk v5 juice

SERVES 1 TO 2

1 medium tomato (6 ounces)

2 cups curly-leaf spinach

½ cup watercress

1 carrot, unpeeled

1 celery rib

⅛–¼ teaspoon Worcestershire sauce (optional)

Coarse sea salt (optional)

why this combination works: Inspired by the ingredient list of commercially available V8—a beverage made up of eight different vegetables—we sought to create a fresh-tasting, lower-sodium vegetable juice. A defining characteristic of V8 is the thick texture of tomato puree, but after trying blanched and canned tomatoes, we opted for a large raw tomato to let its brightly acidic quality shine. This resulted in a more balanced juice where the other vegetables could be tasted equally. Spinach added a vibrant and complex leafy green flavor, while watercress lent pepperiness that worked well with savory celery. And just one carrot provided the right amount of welcome sweetness against the other vegetables in our pared-down ingredient list. Store-bought V8 is quite salty, so in addition to the natural savoriness of juiced celery, we added Worcestershire and sea salt as optional garnishes to our v5 to emulate that flavor without overpowering you with sodium. While tomato is still the primary component of our v5, the concentrated, vibrant green from the spinach and watercress became the predominant color in our homage juice. For more information on processing hearty leafy greens, see page 72. Any variety of tomato will work in this recipe.

On low speed, process tomato through juicer into storage container or serving glass. Increase speed to high and process spinach, watercress, carrot, and celery (in that order). Stir in Worcestershire sauce and sprinkle with salt, if using. Stir to combine before serving.

IF YOU DON'T HAVE

curly-leaf spinach: Use baby spinach.

watercress: Use arugula.

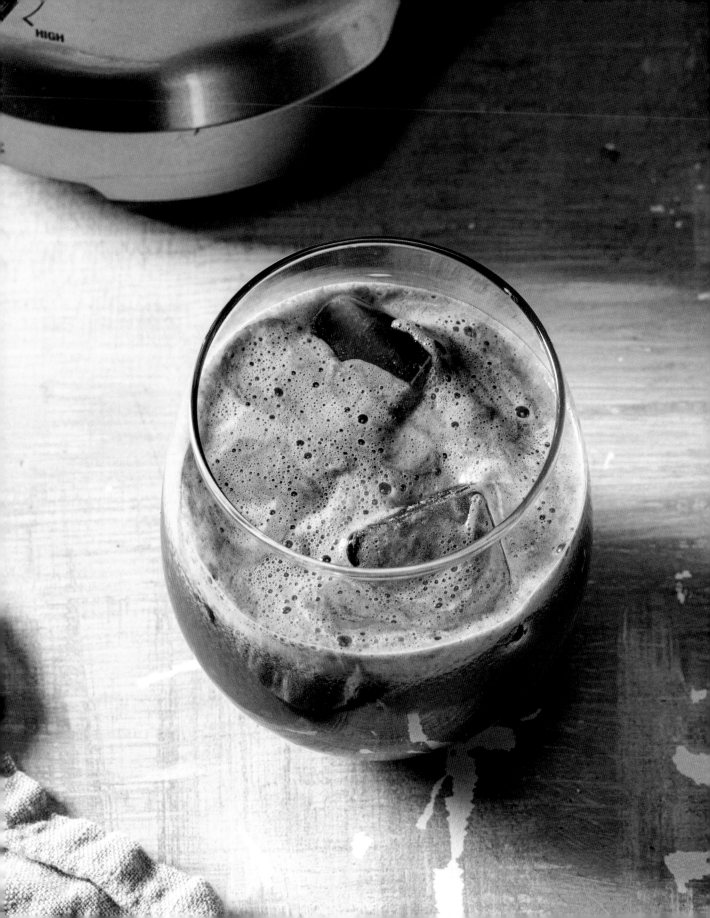

beet sunset juice

SERVES 1 TO 2

1 (1-inch) piece turmeric

5 ounces golden beets, unpeeled, trimmed

4 ounces carrots, unpeeled

6 ounces peeled pineapple

why this combination works: Imagine a tropical sunset, with a gradation of shades from orange to yellow, and then imagine looking into your glass straight from the juicer and tasting something as delightful as it looks. Wanting to exhibit a variety of oranges and yellows through our juicer, we compiled a list of golden ingredients (in quality and color) that would combine to form something greater than the sum of its parts. Golden beets are less sweet and less earthy than their red counterparts, so they ticked our color box while still providing potassium and deep flavor. Carrots were a complementary ingredient to the golden beets because they reinforce each other's pleasant earthy sweetness. We gave the most weight in our drink to tropical pineapple because it carried the theme of our drink while delivering luscious sweetness and a desirable, thickened texture. These three ingredients melded together to form a multifaceted sweet drink that could only be enhanced by our final gold standard ingredient: turmeric. Turmeric delivered a warm, bitter taste that delightfully took the edge off our sweet juice and deepened its background vegetal flavors from the beets and carrots. Be sure to stir your juice before drinking but take time to enjoy the sunset beforehand.

On high speed and in order listed, process all ingredients through juicer into storage container or serving glass. Stir to combine before serving.

IF YOU DON'T HAVE

fresh turmeric: Use ⅛ teaspoon ground turmeric.

golden beets: Use any color beets.

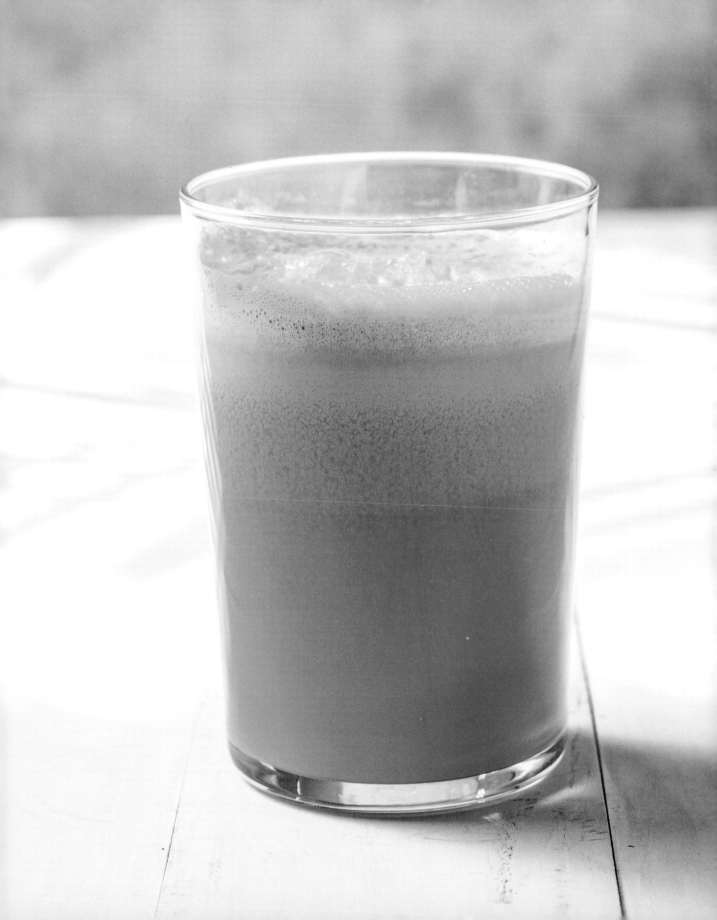

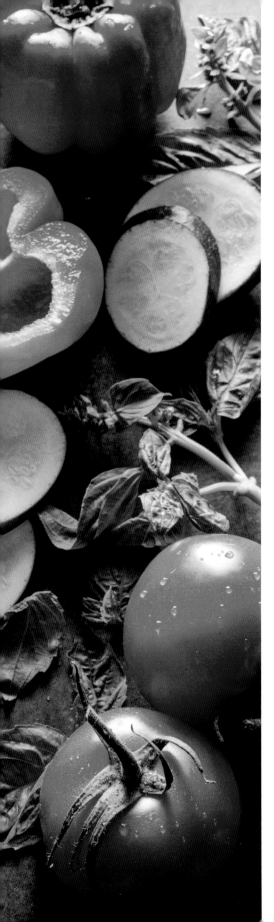
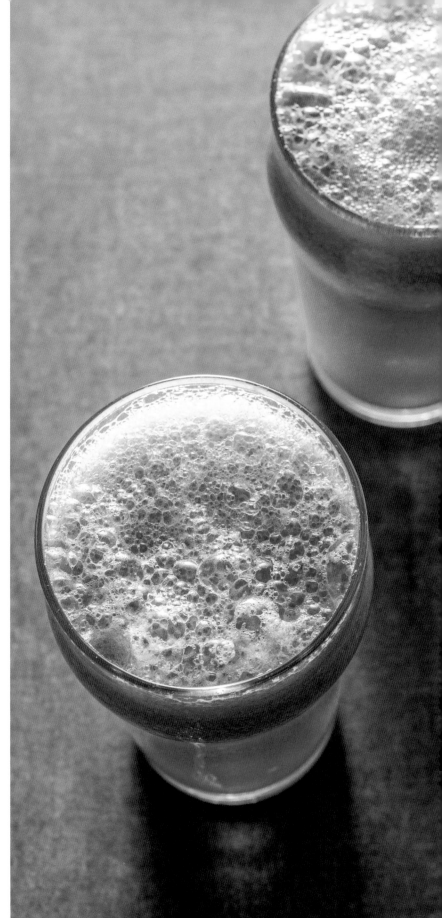

why this combination works: Ever the kitchen experimenters, we wanted to create a juice inspired by the vegetable-laden dish of French ratatouille. Starting with the traditional ingredients of eggplant, bell pepper, zucchini, onion, tomato, and fresh basil, we did some test cook investigating to determine the best combination to translate our inspiration into drinkable form. It turns out that there is a reason people don't juice eggplant, as the taste was too bitter to be palatable; juiced alliums yielded the same unfortunate result. We ended up loving the tomato, zucchini, bell pepper, and basil together, so our juice took on more of a "summer harvest from the garden" theme. The tomato became silky and sugary, the red bell pepper was sweet and vegetal, the zucchini added mostly neutral body, and the fresh basil leaves and stems were herbaceous and savory. The combination will surprise you at first and then compel you to go back for more again and again. Any variety of tomato will work in this recipe.

On low speed, process tomato through juicer into storage container or serving glass. Increase speed to high. In order listed, process remaining ingredients. Stir to combine before serving.

summer garden juice

SERVES 1 TO 2

1 **medium tomato (6 ounces)**

½ **cup fresh basil and tender stems**

½ **red bell pepper, seeded**

½ **zucchini**

IF YOU DON'T HAVE

red bell pepper: Use any color bell pepper.

watermelon salad juice

SERVES 1 TO 2

- **4** **ounces peeled seedless watermelon**

- **4** **ounces romaine lettuce**

- **½** **green bell pepper**

why this combination works: Watermelon is such a sweet and juicy fruit that it can be hard to find suitable pairings. For inspiration we looked to watermelon salads, where savory ingredients like feta cheese and herbs work well with the fruit's sweetness. We knew that red bell pepper made a delicious sweet counterpart in our Watermelon Gazpacho Smoothie (page 30), but here we aimed for a greener and more vegetal taste. Half a green bell pepper brought what we needed; it is less mature than yellow, orange, and red peppers, so it tastes more crisp and verdant. To further our flavor mission, we juiced some romaine lettuce to act as our "salad" base, adding volume and clean flavor. We prefer to use seedless watermelon. Cut your watermelon into the biggest pieces possible that will still fit through the juicing tube in order to yield the most juice. Use whole romaine leaves, leaf side down.

On low speed, process watermelon through juicer into storage container or serving glass. Increase speed to high. In order listed, process remaining ingredients. Stir to combine before serving.

IF YOU DON'T HAVE

watermelon: Use cantaloupe or honeydew.

green bell pepper: Use any color bell pepper.

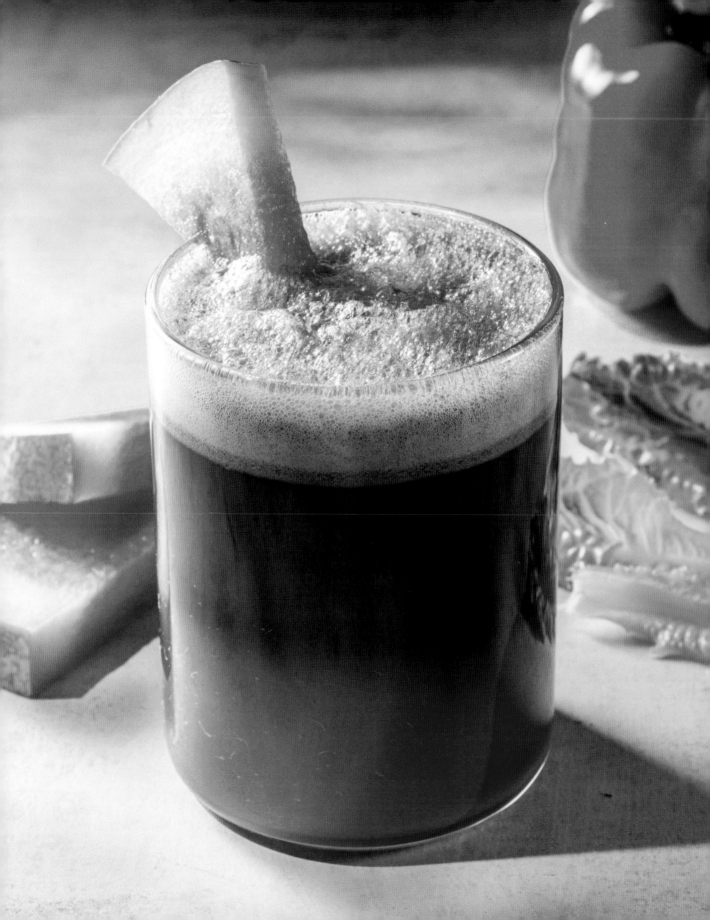

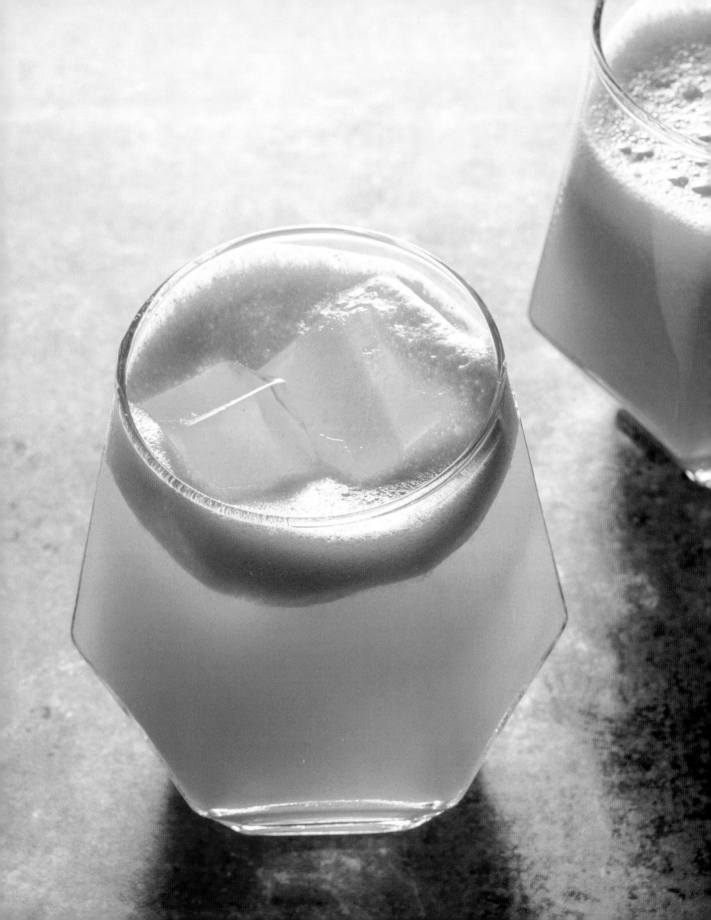

why this combination works: We wanted to use cantaloupe in a juice recipe to harness its tender flesh and sweet flavor, but we also sought to combine it with surprising, punchy additions. Because we drink with our eyes first, we created a vibrant juice that enhanced the cantaloupe's orange color so it would look as good as it tasted. To soften the sweetness of ripe cantaloupe without masking its flavor, we employed yellow summer squash, which provided mild and juicy volume with just a hint of earthiness. That earthiness paired perfectly with the addition of fresh turmeric, which has a neon orange hue and a flavor that is bright, grassy, and a little citrusy. It is not as sharp as other root ingredients like fresh ginger but still imparts a warm spice quality to the juice that was welcome against the fruity cantaloupe and vegetal squash.

On high speed, process turmeric through juicer into storage container or serving glass. Reduce speed to low. In order listed, process remaining ingredients. Stir to combine before serving.

cantaloupe-turmeric juice

SERVES 1 TO 2

- 1 (½-inch) piece turmeric
- 1 large yellow summer squash (10 ounces)
- 6 ounces peeled cantaloupe

IF YOU DON'T HAVE

fresh turmeric: Use pinch of ground turmeric.

yellow summer squash: Use zucchini.

cantaloupe: Use honeydew.

green dream juice

SERVES 1 TO 2

¼ **cup fresh sage leaves and tender stems**

½ **fennel bulb, halved and cored, stalks discarded and fronds reserved**

1 **cup seedless green grapes**

½ **large green apple, cored**

why this combination works: Green Dream sounds like the name of a cocktail—and tastes like one too, with a mixture of fresh ingredients that suggests the herbal flavor of gin without the alcohol. We started on this juice journey wanting to include the vaguely floral quality of fennel for its distinctive anise-like flavor. This fresh licorice hint reminded us of a complex mixed drink, so sweet fruit seemed like a logical addition to round out the juice's profile. Juiced green grapes produced a deliciously sweet nectar with a freshness not found in its syrupy bottled equivalents. Bottled grape juice often contains apple juice, so we took that idea and ran with it: Sticking with our green theme, we added green apple for body and acidic sweetness. We wanted to create a woodsy, herbal taste that paired with the fennel and counteracted the sweetness of our bright fruits, and aromatic sage hit the nail on the head for a juice that has the complexity of a botanical mixed drink. We prefer seedless grapes here. If you can't find fennel with fronds, omit fronds from the recipe.

On low speed, process sage, fennel fronds, and grapes (in that order) through juicer into storage container or serving glass. Increase speed to high and process fennel bulb and apple. Stir to combine before serving.

IF YOU DON'T HAVE

green grapes: Use red grapes.

green apple: Use any color apple.

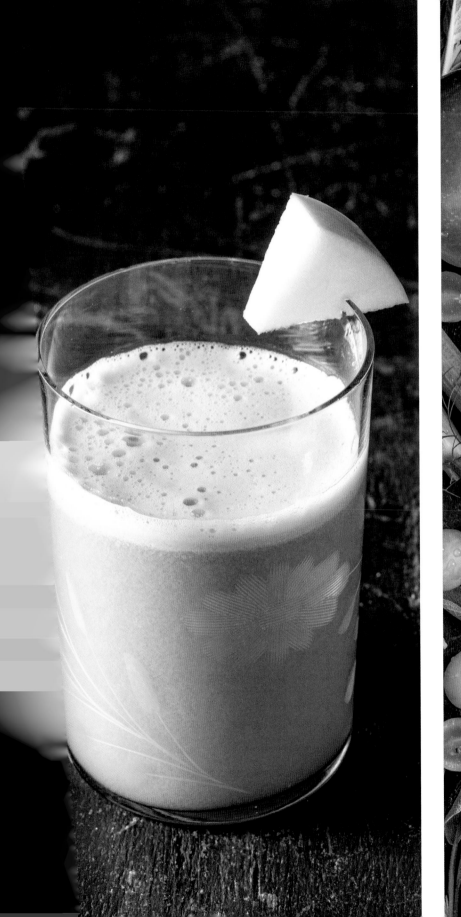
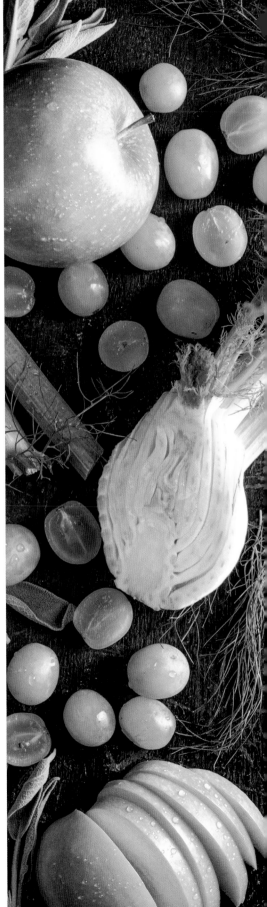

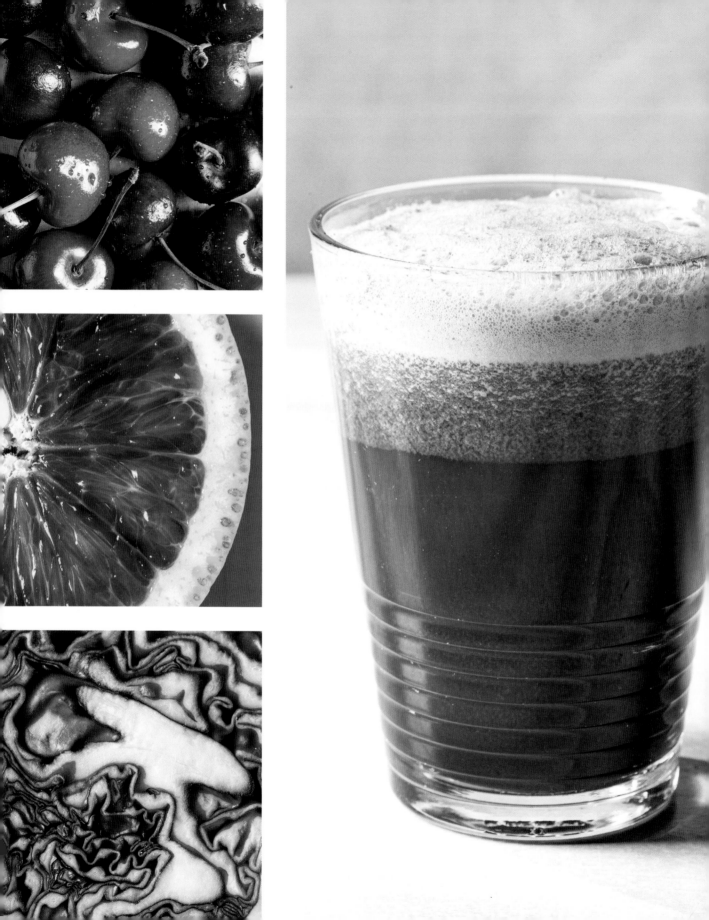

why this combination works: Juicing red cabbage was an astounding discovery because it turned a vivacious purple and had a deep richness that was reminiscent of a Syrah wine, with a distinctly mustardy and peppery flavor. We wanted to add layers of complexity and lean into that almost wine-like flavor without compromising the juice's amazing purple color. Adding sweet cherries for luscious ripeness (plus dark red color) and blood orange for sharp acidic flavor (plus a darker color than other orange varieties) balanced the spiciness of the cabbage and maintained its gorgeous hue. We discovered during testing that the pitted cherries must go into the juicer first so that they don't fly around, splattering you with stains. Follow them quickly with the dense blood orange to weigh them down and extract the most juice. Cut your cabbage into the biggest pieces possible that will still fit through the juicing tube in order to yield the most juice.

On low speed, process cherries and orange (in that order) through juicer into storage container or serving glass. Increase speed to high and process cabbage. Stir to combine before serving.

can't believe there's cabbage juice

SERVES 1 TO 2

- **5 ounces fresh sweet cherries, pitted**
- **1 blood orange, peeled**
- **9 ounces red cabbage**

IF YOU DON'T HAVE

fresh cherries: Use thawed frozen cherries.

blood orange: Use navel orange.

sweet potato– cranberry juice

SERVES 1 TO 2

1 (¼-inch-thick) slice orange

⅓ cup cranberries

1 medium sweet potato (12 ounces), unpeeled and halved lengthwise

Pinch ground cinnamon (optional)

IF YOU DON'T HAVE

cranberries: Use thawed frozen cranberries.

why this combination works: Sweet potato, cranberries, a slice of orange, and a pinch of cinnamon make up this Thanksgiving-inspired juice. Sweet potato served as the backdrop for this exciting drink because it created a mildly sweet canvas to build upon, and the starch from the potato added body and slight texture to the juice. Cranberries, while not typically consumed raw because they are so tart, were mellowed in the creamy sweet potato juice and added a bright pop of acidity. Just one slice of orange bridged the tang of the cranberries and the sweetness of the sweet potato with a hint of acidic citrus that still allowed the dominant flavors to come through. A final pinch of warm cinnamon was a divisive choice among tasters, with half loving it and half choosing to pass, but it can be added to make this juice distinctly autumnal.

On low speed, process orange through juicer into storage container or serving glass. Increase speed to high and process cranberries and potato (in that order). Stir in cinnamon, if using. Stir to combine before serving.

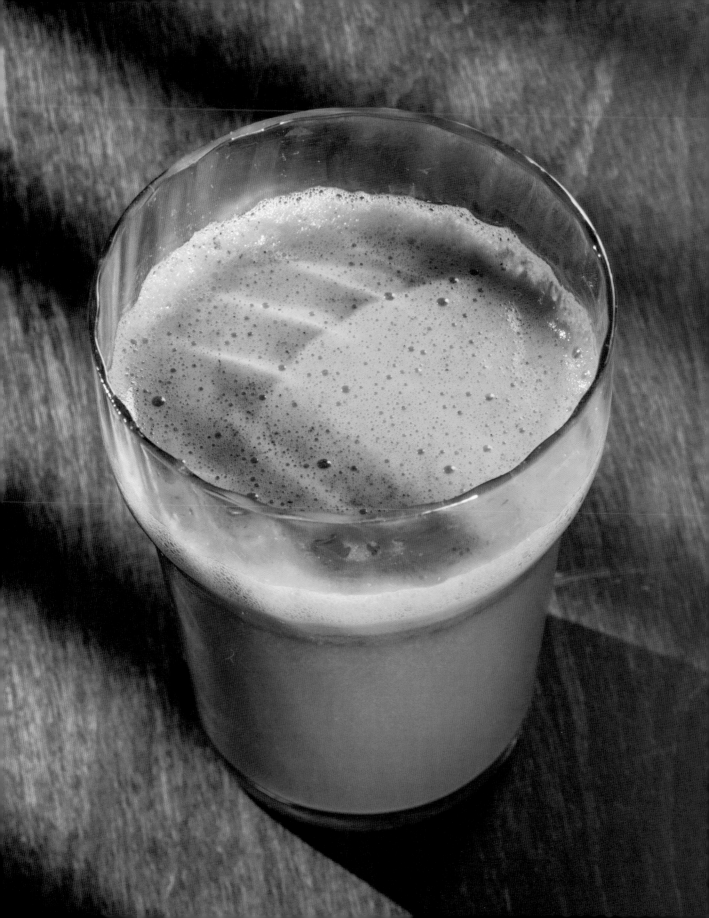

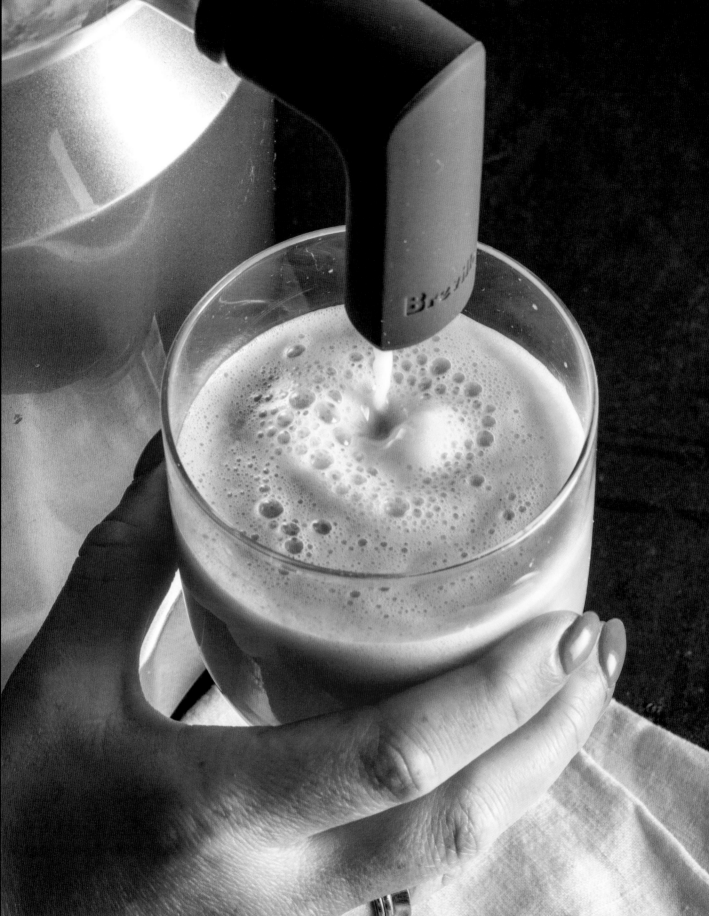

why this combination works: While you might be skeptical at the thought of juicing a parsnip, its unique taste evokes flavors of sweet potatoes and warm spices that make for a delicious base. Here, the starchy and sweet parsnip was complemented by a ripe, juicy pear as both are surprisingly sweet and thick, which produced a juice with solid body. Unfortunately, pale parsnips and a pear do not make for a pretty pair color-wise. When looking for a colorful add-in, we tasted regular oranges versus blood oranges; the latter provided a much-needed, berry-like tartness that mellowed out the sweetness of the juice—and contributed a vibrant fuchsia hue. For a little zip, fresh ginger invigorated and enlivened the entire combination. Look for parsnips that are firm, with a carrot-like snap, and less tapered and more uniform in size, as these contain more of the sweet vegetable flesh and less bitter root core.

On high speed, process ginger and parsnips (in that order) through juicer into storage container or serving glass. Reduce speed to low and process orange and pear (in that order). Stir to combine before serving.

parsnip and pear juice

SERVES 1 TO 2

1 (½-inch) piece ginger

6 ounces parsnips, unpeeled

½ blood orange, peeled

1 ripe but firm pear, halved and cored

IF YOU DON'T HAVE

blood orange: Use navel orange.

teas, tisanes & more

teas 101

Perhaps the most universal beverage, tea is a vast category. Hot or cold, bagged or loose, herbal or astringent, the possibilities are endless and can feel overwhelming. We wanted to develop a wide range of hot teas, cold teas, tisanes, and dried blends with inspiration from around the world to help you delve into tea making and more. Tisanes are herbal tea infusions that can be served hot or cold, and are fragrant and flavorful—just try our Hibiscus Iced Tea (page 131). And while tea is a beverage itself, we also treated it as an ingredient within recipes like Cha Manao (page 128), which uses loose-leaf Assam alongside warm spices and lime juice. Whether you want to entertain guests or soothe an upset stomach, we experimented with every variable possible from temperature and time to quantity and quality to give you top-tier recipes.

brewing

WHAT TO USE

Electric, stovetop, and gooseneck kettles all have one thing in common: Any of them can make tea. Even a pot of boiling water will do. And while some pieces of≈equipment might be easier to use than others, the most important factor to ensure the quality of your tea is getting the right temperature. We found that even a few degrees difference can greatly impact the quality of your result, so it is essential that you take the temperature of your water. If your kettle doesn't allow you to set the temperature automatically, see our Tea Drinker's Toolkit on page 123 for specifics on a thermometer. For information about our kettle buying recommendations, see page 11.

WHAT TO KNOW

Throughout the chapter, we implement many different brewing and steeping methods depending upon the desired end result. Sometimes we simmer delicate teas and aromatic compounds to gently meld their flavors together before chilling. Other times we employ a traditional hot steeping method (with the temperature and strength dependent upon the tea type and amount) to optimally extract flavorful compounds. When experimenting with iced teas, we discovered that traditional cold brewing methods can overextract the tea and result in a murky and bitter drink. To remedy this, we developed a hybrid method. We started by steeping the tea in boiling water for several minutes before adding ice water and steeping for another hour. This method works to pull out the strong flavors of the tea before allowing it to gently infuse at a lower temperature over the course of an hour. To ensure success, your ice water should always be half ice and half water. For an accurate measurement of boiling water, bring a kettle of water to a boil and then measure out the desired amount.

what's the difference between teas?

Much of the variation between teas has to do with how the leaves are processed after harvesting. When tea leaves are picked, they rapidly start to undergo chemical changes. Many varieties of tea can actually be made from the same plant. Oxidation causes the green leaves to turn deep reddish-brown and develop typical tea flavors, including astringency. To make black tea, the leaves are often rolled, cut, or crushed, and/or held at warm temperatures, all of which encourage those reactions. To make green tea, the objective is to prevent the reactions, so the leaves stay green and the flavor more delicate. As soon as possible after harvest, the leaves' enzymes are deactivated with a blast of heat. That preserves many flavor compounds that would otherwise be transformed or destroyed, including amino acids that give green tea its umami savor. White tea is harvested younger than the other teas, and minimally oxidized, so it's typically even more delicate than green tea.

LOOSE-LEAF VERSUS BAGGED TEA

The biggest difference between loose-leaf teas and their bagged counterparts is their size and quality. Loose-leaf teas contain bigger, more intact pieces, whereas bagged tea is typically composed of smaller, more broken pieces of that same tea—yet both have their place. We almost always prefer loose-leaf tea for its higher quality. However, bagged teas can make a perfectly acceptable alternative to loose-leaf teas, especially when combined with other flavors in iced teas (see pages 124–131).

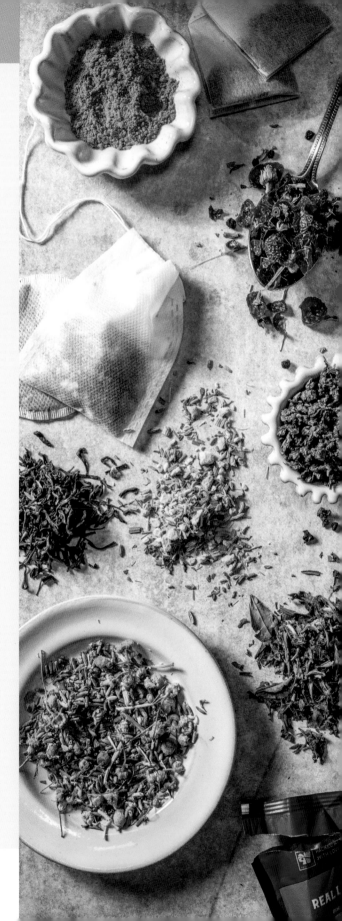

tea, times & temperatures

Here are the basic formulas for brewing different varieties of tea with amounts per 1-cup serving. Times at the end of a steep range will produce a stronger cup of tea. This is beneficial in drinks such as London Fog Tea Latte (page 136), where the flavor will be diluted. Steep times may vary by blend, so pay attention to your brand's packaging and follow specific recipe instructions closely.

TEA TYPE	TEMPERATURE	STEEP TIME	NOTES
black tea *1 teaspoon*	212 degrees	3 to 5 minutes	For iced black tea, if you use too much tea it becomes cloudy from caffeine and tannins.
white tea *2 teaspoons*	180 to 185 degrees	4 to 5 minutes	White tea leaves are more delicate and therefore less dense and compact, so they require a larger quantity than other tea types.
Earl Grey tea *1 teaspoon*	208 degrees	3 to 5 minutes	At 212 degrees, the boiling water worked to pull out too much citrus oil from the bergamot, which left the tea overly bitter. 208 degrees ended up being the perfect temperature to ensure a flavorful, drinkable tea.
green tea *1 teaspoon*	175 degrees	3 to 5 minutes	Green tea leaves are not oxidized like black leaves, so you should never use boiling water as it will burn the leaves and taint the flavor profile.
gunpowder green tea *1 teaspoon*	212 degrees	An initial rinse, then drain and steep for 5 to 6 minutes	Gunpowder green tea is rinsed with boiling water to help wash away particulates and bitterness before steeping.
herbal tea blend *1 tablespoon*	212 degrees	10 minutes	A 5-minute steep was watery, lacking flavor, and underextracted. A 15-minute steep cooled down too quickly before drinking and overextracted the compounds.
herbal tea blend with chamomile *1 tablespoon*	212 degrees	5 to 7 minutes	When chamomile was present in blends, it required less steeping time because it became overextracted and bitter.

keys to a foolproof cup of tea

CHECK WATER QUALITY
If your tap water is hard, it has lots of mineral deposits that can compromise the flavor of your tea—run it through a filter, or use bottled water instead.

ADJUST WATER TEMPERATURE
Ensure your water is the correct temperature by using an automatic kettle that can set the temperature or by using a simple thermometer.

DON'T OVERSTEEP
The longer you steep, the more tannins will leach out of the leaves, making your infusion bitter and overwhelming the tea's more delicate flavors. Pay attention to your packaging's recommended times and check out our tea time chart (see page 120).

BONUS!
make multiple infusions: You can reuse the same tea leaves for multiple cups. For a second or third infusion, you'll simply want to increase the steeping time, tasting as you go until you arrive at a flavor you like.

tips to mix and match your own dried blends

Now that you understand the varying brew times and their relevant factors, we encourage you to make your own dried tea blends. We have examples (see pages 147–154), but there are some things to keep in mind when combining flavors and elements to create your own custom teas.

- Citrus-forward flavors pair well with strong black teas.

- For herbal blends, start by focusing on the health aspect that you want to create, then taste ingredients individually to home in on a unique flavor profile and find a balance of bitter, floral, warm spiced, and bright citrus notes.

- The shape and size of certain dried elements matter. For dried ingredients where you want more infusion, expose more surface area by putting them into a spice grinder or by using a mortar and pestle to break them into smaller pieces.

WHAT IS ASSAM?
Have you ever wondered what exactly Assam tea is? It is a particular type of black tea produced in the Assam region of India. Due to its naturally high caffeine content, Assam tea is frequently marketed as a breakfast tea and, in fact, many Irish and English breakfast teas use Assam or a blend that includes it. The tea is described as having a rich, savory aroma and a malty finish.

making the perfect matcha

We spent a lot of time and effort in the kitchen using customary methods and equipment to deliver a deliciously drinkable tea. Here we break down the key factors that contribute to making the perfect cup of matcha.

PAY ATTENTION TO THE MATCHA GRADE

There are three grades of matcha: ceremonial, premium, and culinary. Ceremonial and premium grades are made to consume as a tea or latte, and the former is traditionally used for important ceremonies. You can substitute premium grade for ceremonial, but culinary-grade matcha is used solely in cooking and should not be made into a drink.

EQUIPMENT CAN IMPACT FLAVOR

We discovered that the use of a traditional chawan and chasen (tea bowl and whisk) creates a smoother, creamier beverage with a much thicker, delicate foam. We encourage you to take part in this tradition; however, a small ceramic or glass soup bowl and small whisk or a milk frother can be used. See Frothing Milk at Home for more information.

TEMPERATURE IS CRITICAL

175 degrees is the traditional recommended temperature for matcha. When brewed with water below 175, the matcha did not suspend as well into the water. This concept is unique to matcha because the tea isn't strained; it is whisked and suspended into the final drink when it dissolves.

Chasen and chawan: A chasen is a traditional bamboo whisk used to aerate matcha, and a chawan is the accompanying bowl/cup, which is larger than a normal cup to accommodate the whisking inside before drinking from it.

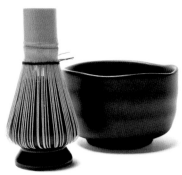

FROTHING MILK AT HOME

While frothed milk can seem like a coffeehouse luxury, it is easy to obtain at home, even if you don't have any special equipment. We tested four methods: hand whisking, blending, immersion blending, and jar shaking. Milk frothing worked well with all methods for all dairy and plant-based milk options, except for soy milk, which required the strength of a handheld immersion blender to whip up. All methods of whisking were successful and can be used, but we preferred the simplicity and accessibility of hand whisking. Note that milk options need to be heated to 140 to 155 degrees before frothing. See our Tea Drinker's Toolkit on page 123 for information on our preferred whisk.

tea drinker's toolkit

While no piece of equipment is absolutely essential to tea making, these items can certainly help.

THERMOMETER

We turn to a digital thermometer to help ensure the accuracy of our water's temperature, as this is the most important factor in brewing high-quality tea. Our winning thermometer is the **Thermapen ONE**.

MINI WHISK

For accessible milk frothing, we recommend using a small, compact whisk and a bowl of your choosing. Our winner is the **Tovolo Stainless Steel 6" Mini Whisk**.

MILK FROTHER

A handheld frother is a less labor-intensive way to froth milk. Our winner is the lightweight and powerful **Zulay Kitchen Milk Boss Electric Milk Frother**.

TEA INFUSER

Tea infusers are great for making a single cup of loose-leaf tea. You simply measure the amount of tea you want to use into the infuser, stick the infuser into a cup, and pour hot water over it. Our winner is the **Finum Brewing Basket L**.

TEA SACHET

These mesh bags are great for making a single cup of loose-leaf tea. Simply stuff the sachet with your desired amount of tea and use it the same way you would a store-bought tea bag.

BAGGED TEA

Bagged tea can sometimes be a perfectly viable substitute for loose-leaf tea. See the recipe specifics for how many bags to use. Our winning black teas are **Twinings English Breakfast Tea** and **Tetley British Blend**, and our winning green tea is **Celestial Seasonings Authentic Green Tea**.

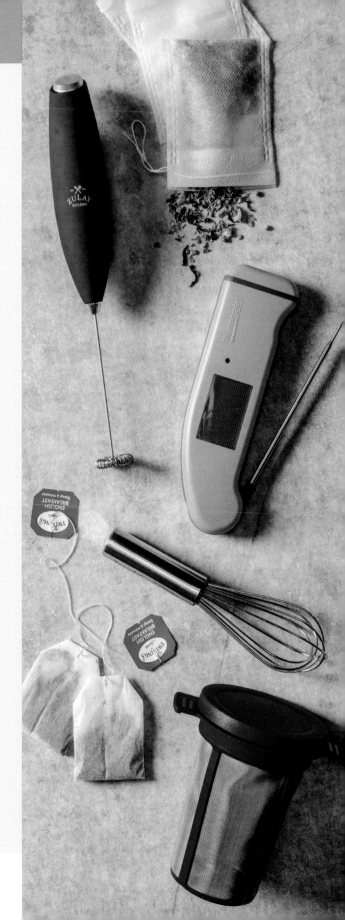

iced black tea

SERVES 4

1½ tablespoons black tea leaves

3 cups boiling water

1 cup ice water

Lemon wedges

IF YOU DON'T HAVE

loose-leaf black tea: Use 2 tea bags.

why this combination works: We made our own brisk and refreshing iced tea so we could control the intensity of the flavor (and the sugar amount). When we compared iced teas made from loose-leaf tea versus tea bags, we found the former produced a more flavorful, complex drink. Conversely, when we tested our flavored variations with loose and bagged tea, the differences were too subtle to necessitate using loose-leaf only. Iced tea can be brewed using either cold or boiling water, but we found that a cold-infused tea tasted flat, and boiling water made bitter, mouth-drying tea. We ultimately devised a technique that produced balanced flavor by combining the two methods. First, we steeped the tea in water that had been brought to a boil, then added ice water and continued to steep for an hour. At the cooler temperature, the aromatic compounds infused the water, while the bitter and astringent ones did not. The final tea can be enjoyed as is or sweetened to taste with homemade Simple Syrup (page 5). Both caffeinated and decaffeinated tea work well here. This recipe can easily be doubled.

Place tea in medium bowl. Add boiling water and steep for 4 minutes. Add ice water and steep for 1 hour. Strain through fine-mesh strainer into pitcher or large container (or strain into second bowl and transfer to pitcher). Refrigerate until chilled, at least 1 hour or up to 3 days. Serve in ice-filled glasses, garnished with lemon wedges.

VARIATIONS
raspberry-basil iced black tea
Omit lemon. Mash 1½ cups thawed frozen raspberries, 3 tablespoons chopped fresh basil, 2 tablespoons sugar, and 2 teaspoons lemon juice in bowl until no whole berries remain. Add mixture to tea with ice water. Garnish each serving with basil sprig.

ginger-pomegranate iced black tea
Add ⅔ cup pomegranate juice, 2 tablespoons sugar, and 1½ to 2 tablespoons grated fresh ginger to tea with ice water. Substitute lime wedges for lemon.

apple-cinnamon iced black tea
Omit lemon. Add ½ cinnamon stick to medium bowl with tea. Add 1 cored and shredded red apple and 1 tablespoon sugar to tea with ice water.

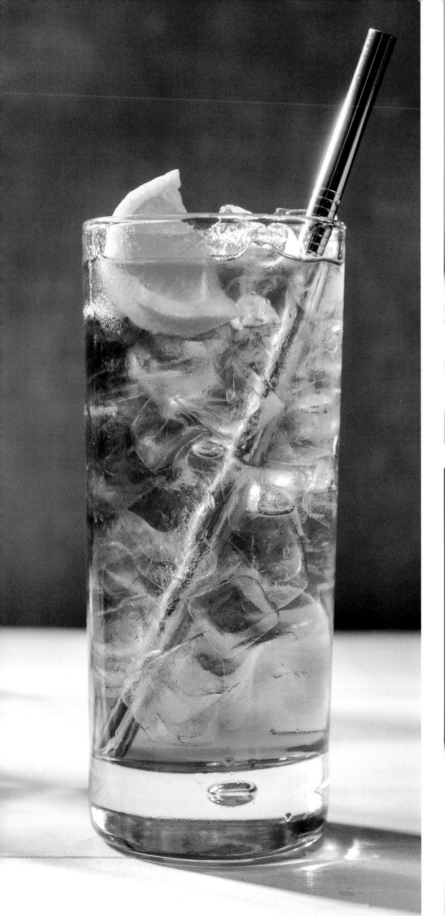
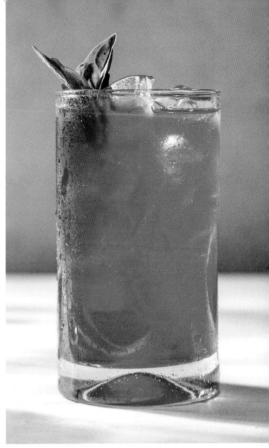
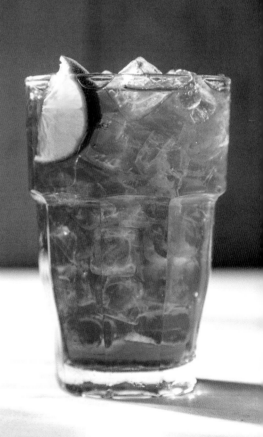

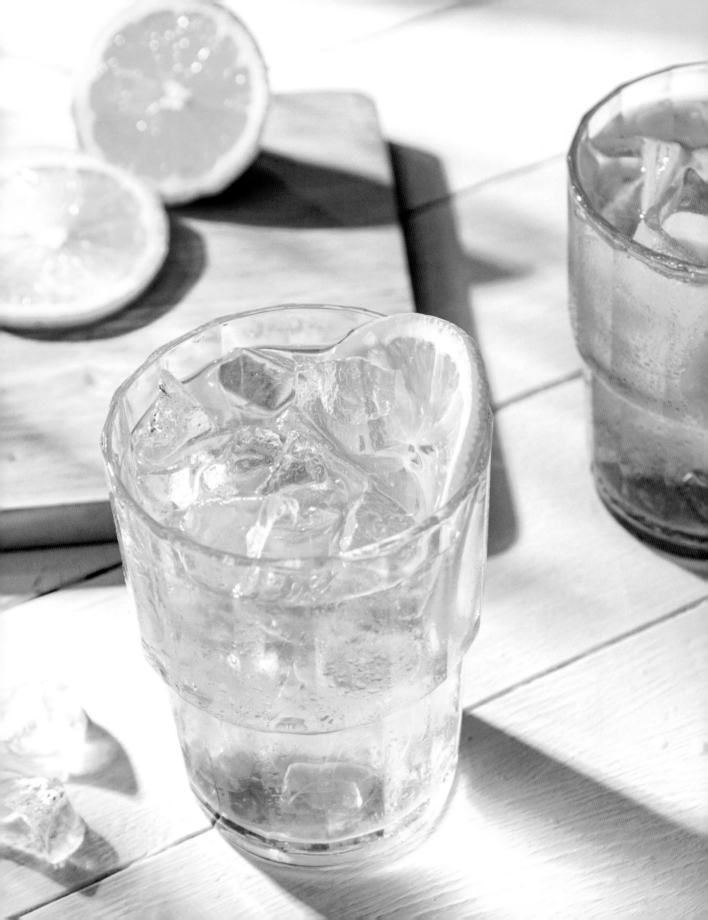

why this combination works: A widely consumed drink around the world (and especially throughout Asia), green tea is earthy and invigorating and, when made correctly, never bitter. For iced green tea, we employed the same method used in our Iced Black Tea (page 124) but with the temperatures adjusted so as to not over-extract the more sensitive tea leaves. To get a green tea that was smooth and mellow, we started by brewing tea with 175-degree water. Then we cooled the extraction but did not strain it. By steeping the tea for an hour at this lower temperature, we could slowly draw more delicate flavor from the leaves. This resulted in a smooth, drinkable iced tea that is perfect alone but can also be enhanced with unique flavor pairings such as the refreshing cantaloupe-mint or the elevated pear and sage variations. Chinese green tea will produce a grassy, floral tea, whereas Japanese green tea is more savory. The final tea can be enjoyed as is or sweetened to taste with homemade Simple Syrup (page 5). Both caffeinated and decaffeinated loose-leaf tea work well here. This recipe can easily be doubled.

Place tea in medium bowl. Add hot water and steep for 4 minutes. Add ice water and steep for 1 hour. Strain through fine-mesh strainer into pitcher or large container (or strain into second bowl and transfer to pitcher). Refrigerate until chilled, at least 1 hour or up to 3 days. Serve in ice-filled glasses, garnished with lemon wedges.

VARIATIONS

cantaloupe-mint iced green tea
Omit lemon. Add 1 cup grated cantaloupe pulp, 3 tablespoons chopped fresh mint, 2 tablespoons sugar, and 1 tablespoon lemon juice to tea with ice water. Garnish each serving with mint sprig.

cucumber-lime iced green tea
Shred ½ English cucumber on large holes of box grater. Add shredded cucumber, 2 tablespoons sugar, ½ teaspoon grated lime zest, and 1 tablespoon lime juice to tea with ice water. Substitute lime slices for lemon wedges.

pear-sage iced green tea
Omit lemon. Add 1 cored and shredded pear, 2 tablespoons sugar, and 1 teaspoon minced fresh sage to tea with ice water.

iced green tea

SERVES 4

2 **tablespoons green tea leaves**

3 **cups hot water (175 degrees)**

1 **cup ice water**

Lemon wedges

IF YOU DON'T HAVE

loose-leaf green tea: Use 2 tea bags.

cha manao

SERVES 4

1½ tablespoons Assam tea leaves

1 tablespoon annatto seeds

1 cinnamon stick

2 star anise pods

¼ cup sugar

4 cups boiling water

1½ teaspoons vanilla extract

3 tablespoons lime juice

Lime wedges (optional)

IF YOU DON'T HAVE

Assam tea: Use English or Irish breakfast tea.

why this combination works: Cha manao, sometimes spelled in other ways, translates to "lime tea" and is a Thai iced tea. It is steeped with spices and a red coloring agent and then sweetened and served with lime juice. The backbone of this drink comes from loose-leaf Assam tea because it lends a delicate, not overly bitter flavor when compared to bagged tea. Thai tea blends contain a wide range of warm spices, so we chose cinnamon and star anise, as they were common throughout homemade blends and imparted earthy spiced notes. To keep the red color that is characteristic of Thai tea while avoiding unnatural food dyes, we opted to use annatto seeds. Whole annatto seeds gave us a deep red color without much added flavor, and they didn't leave the tea cloudy or gritty like powdered annatto did. Vanilla extract provided flavor without any additional sweetness, while lime juice—the most readily available citrus in Thailand—gave our cha manao its distinctively refreshing flavor. It was important to keep the sweet-sour balance appropriately strong as this is key to the identity of cha manao, so we still included some sugar and added the lime juice just before serving to preserve its fresh and vibrant qualities. This resulted in an iced tea that was lightly sweetened and delicately spiced with a nice, acidic kick.

1. Place tea, annatto seeds, cinnamon stick, star anise, and sugar in medium bowl. Add boiling water and stir to dissolve sugar. Steep for 4 minutes. Strain through fine-mesh strainer into pitcher or large container (or strain into second bowl and transfer to pitcher). Stir in vanilla. Refrigerate until chilled, at least 1 hour or up to 3 days.

2. Just before serving, stir lime juice into tea. Pour into ice-filled glasses and garnish with lime wedges, if using. (To make a single portion, combine 1 cup tea and 2 teaspoons juice in glass before adding ice.)

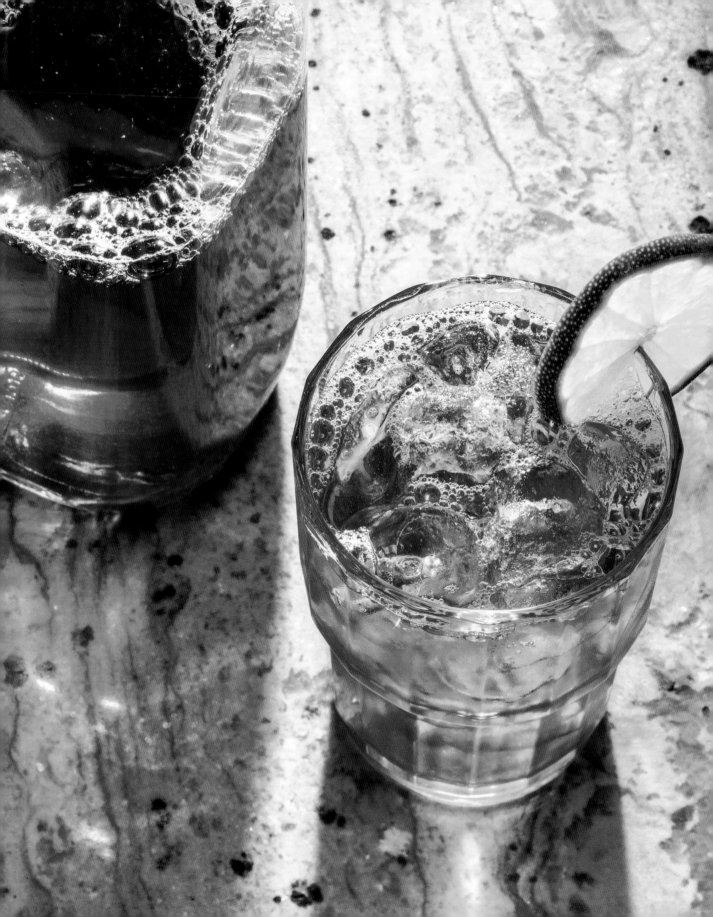

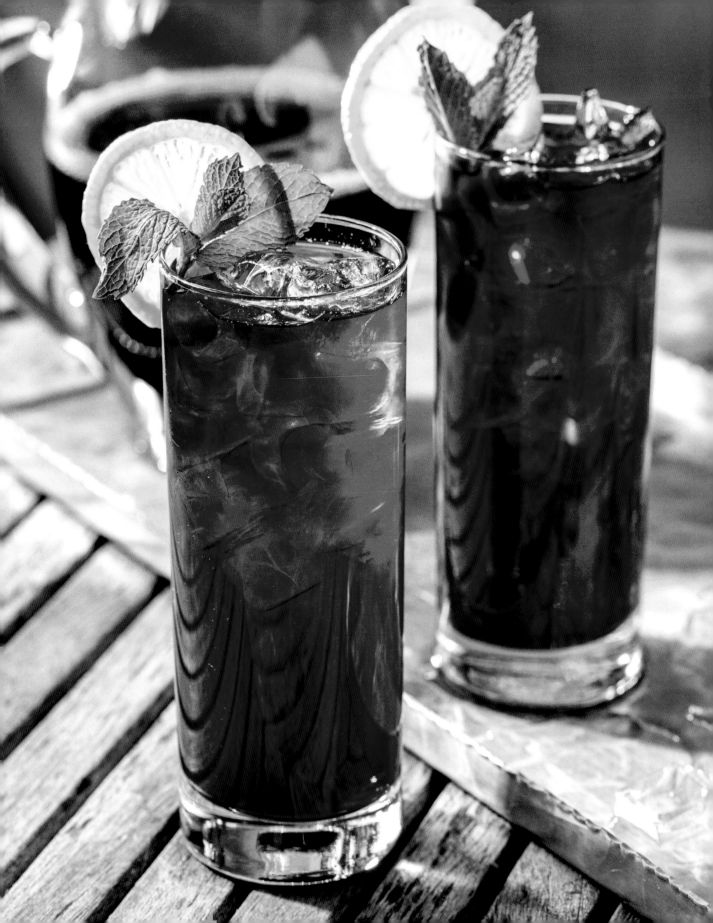

why this combination works: Hibiscus teas have roots in West Africa and have long been incorporated into Juneteenth celebrations in the United States. West Africans used their native plant hibiscus, also known as roselle, to make a popular hospitality drink called bissap. Sweeteners, such as cane syrup, as well as fragrant, bright-tasting citrus, ginger, and other spices, were added to balance the bitterness. In this recipe, created by mixologist Tiffanie Barriere, we steeped whole dried hibiscus flowers with orange, lemon, ginger, cinnamon, clove, and star anise for a traditional and tasty infusion. We avoided letting the tea boil, as that can make it too bitter, and instead let it gently simmer for 20 minutes. We then strained out the solids, let the tea cool, and added cane syrup for sweetness (you can add more to taste if you like a slightly sweeter tea). Use whole dried hibiscus flowers, not ones that have been cut and sifted. If you can find only ones that have been cut and sifted, use the weight listed (1½ ounces), not the volume. This recipe can easily be doubled.

1. Bring water, hibiscus flowers, orange zest and juice, lemon zest and juice, ginger, cinnamon stick, star anise, and clove to simmer in large saucepan over medium heat. Reduce heat to low and steep until mixture is fragrant and flavors meld, about 20 minutes.

2. Strain mixture through fine-mesh strainer into large bowl or storage container. Refrigerate until chilled, at least 1 hour or up to 10 days.

3. Transfer strained tea to serving pitcher and stir in cane syrup. Serve in ice-filled glasses.

hibiscus iced tea

SERVES 4 TO 6

6 cups water

1½ ounces whole dried hibiscus flowers (about 1½ cups)

6 (3-inch) strips orange zest plus 2 tablespoons juice

6 (2-inch) strips lemon zest plus 2 tablespoons juice

1 (½-inch) piece ginger, peeled and sliced thin

1 cinnamon stick

1 star anise pod

1 whole clove

2–4 tablespoons cane syrup

cold brew coffee concentrate

SERVES 4
(MAKES ABOUT 4 CUPS)

8 ounces medium-roast coffee beans, ground coarse (3 cups)

4 cups filtered water, room temperature

Kosher salt (optional)

IF YOU DON'T HAVE

medium-roast coffee beans:
Use light or dark roast.

why this combination works: Cold brew has mild acidity and bitterness that lets more of the subtle, hidden flavors of coffee come through. With regular coffee brewed hot, the heat works to extract bitterness and astringency from the beans. Here, we used common household equipment for our steep (a 2-quart Mason jar, strainer, and coffee filter) so that the recipe is accessible to any coffee drinker. Using a high ratio of ground beans to water produced a concentrate that was easy to store and could be diluted as desired. Double straining the concentrate ensured our drink was free of sediment. Our finishing touch was a pinch of kosher salt, which rounded out the cold brew's flavors. This concentrate needs to be diluted before drinking. We recommend a 1:1 ratio of concentrate to water, but you can dilute it more if you like.

1. Stir coffee and water together in 2-quart jar or narrow pitcher. Allow raft of ground coffee to form, about 10 minutes, then stir again to recombine. Cover with plastic wrap and let steep at room temperature for 24 hours.

2. Set fine-mesh strainer over large bowl. Pour concentrate into strainer and using back of ladle or rubber spatula, gently stir concentrate to help filter through strainer, extracting as much liquid as possible. Discard grounds.

3. Set now-empty strainer over second large bowl and line with large coffee filter. Strain concentrate for a second time through prepared strainer, gently stirring concentrate to help filter through strainer. (This may take up to 10 minutes). Transfer to airtight container. Refrigerate until chilled, at least 1 hour or up to 1 week.

to make iced coffee: Add ½ cup coffee concentrate, ½ cup cold water, and pinch kosher salt, if using, to ice-filled glass. Gently stir to combine.

VARIATIONS
pumpkin-spiced cold brew coffee concentrate
Add 2 teaspoons toasted and cracked allspice berries, 4 toasted and cracked cinnamon sticks, and 12 toasted whole cloves to coffee and water mixture in step 1.

star anise—orange cold brew coffee concentrate
Add 1 toasted star anise pod and 1 tablespoon grated orange zest to coffee and water mixture in step 1.

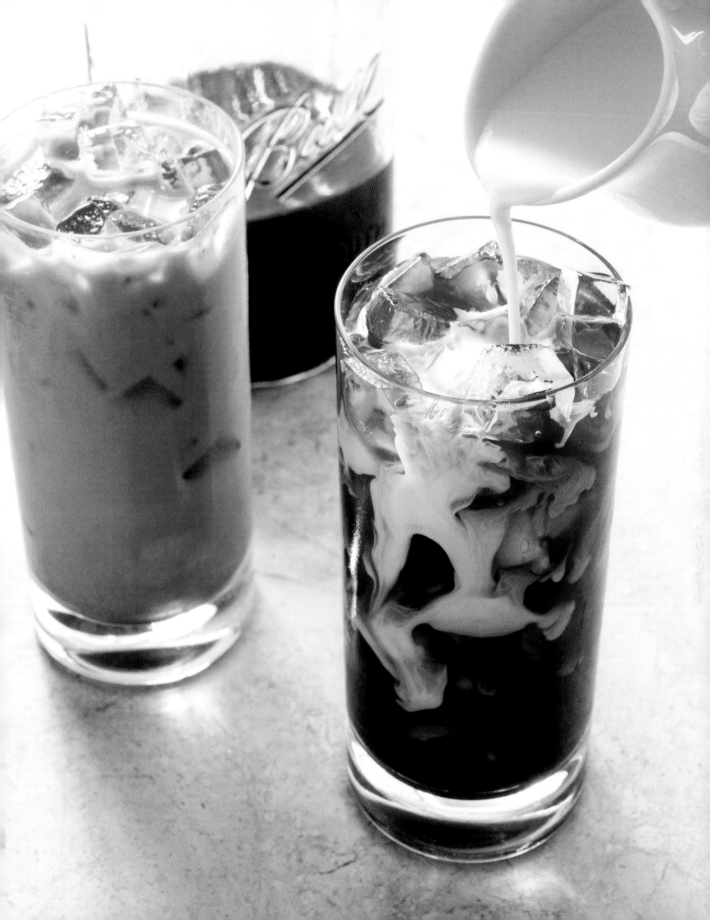

masala chai concentrate

SERVES 6
(MAKES ABOUT 4 CUPS)

3 cinnamon sticks

1 star anise pod

15 green cardamom pods

2 teaspoons whole cloves

¾ teaspoon black peppercorns

5 cups water

¼ cup packed brown sugar

1 tablespoon finely chopped fresh ginger

Pinch table salt

3 tablespoons black tea leaves

why this combination works: Masala chai, which originated in India but has gained popularity around the world, is a sweet and milky spiced tea that can be enjoyed hot or cold. It has the flavor of black tea combined with milk, sugar, and a lengthy list of warm spices. To avoid sediment in our tea, we crushed the spices rather than grind them before toasting because it resulted in bigger pieces rather than a powder. We simmered cinnamon, star anise, cardamom, cloves, and black peppercorns in water for a full 10 minutes before adding the tea leaves. This ensured that the potent spices' lively flavors would hold their own against a strong black tea extraction. We combined the spices with caramelly brown sugar and fresh, invigorating ginger, which mellowed in the hot water but was still plenty punchy. The resulting concentrate was sweet, spiced, and bracing enough to stand up to plenty of milk for a balanced masala chai at whatever temperature you prefer. A boldly flavored tea such as Assam is ideal for this recipe; alternatively, use Irish or English breakfast tea. To avoid dusty sediment in the tea, be sure to crush (not grind) the spices before toasting them. If you have one, a mortar and pestle can be used to crush the spices.

1. Place cinnamon sticks and star anise on cutting board. Using back of heavy skillet, press down firmly until spices are coarsely crushed; transfer to medium saucepan. Crush cardamom pods, cloves, and peppercorns and add to saucepan. Toast spices over medium heat, stirring frequently, until fragrant, 1 to 2 minutes.

2. Add water, sugar, ginger, and salt and bring to boil. Cover saucepan, reduce heat, and simmer mixture for 10 minutes. Stir in tea, cover, and simmer for 10 minutes. Remove from heat and let tea and spices steep for 10 minutes. Strain mixture through fine-mesh strainer. Refrigerate until chilled, at least 1 hour or up to 1 week. Stir before using.

to make hot masala chai: Stir ½ cup concentrate and ½ cup milk together in saucepan and heat to desired temperature, or combine in mug and heat in microwave.

to make iced masala chai: Add ⅔ cup concentrate and ⅓ cup milk to ice-filled glass. Gently stir to combine.

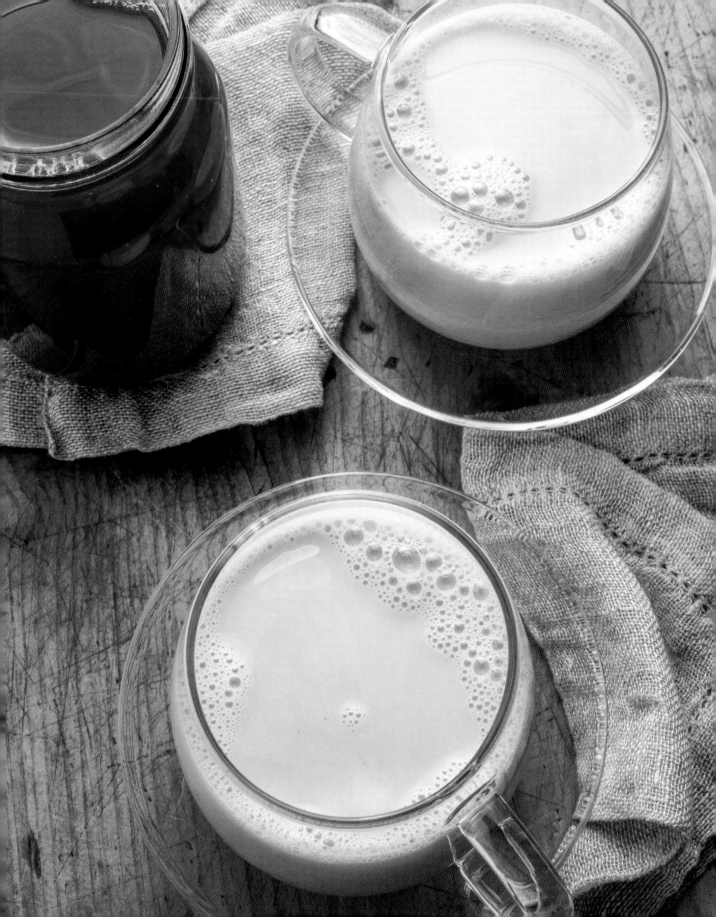

london fog tea latte

SERVES 1

1½ teaspoons Earl Grey tea leaves

1 green cardamom pod, cracked

½ cup hot water (208 degrees)

½ cup dairy or plant-based milk

¼–½ teaspoon vanilla extract

why this combination works: As taken as we are by the London Fog drink, which consists of Earl Grey tea, steamed milk, and sweetened vanilla syrup, we wanted to enjoy it as a hot latte without the added sugar. Bergamot is a lime-looking but orange-tasting citrus fruit native to Italy, and it's the ingredient in Earl Grey tea that gives it such a distinctive flavor. That citrus oil provides a floral complexity to the tea, so we combined two potent spices to complement that floral nature: rich vanilla extract and aromatic cardamom pods. The vanilla provided sweet flavor without the additional sweetness, while cardamom pods gave the tea an earthy-spiced note. To turn this drink into a latte, we preferred the simplicity of a saucepan and a whisk to create our steamed milk, but any method will do. Any type of dairy or nondairy milk will work here; soy milk will yield less foam, so we recommend using an immersion blender.

1. Add tea and cardamom pod to tea infuser or tea sachet. Steep tea mixture with hot water in teacup, covered, for 5 minutes.

2. Meanwhile, heat milk and vanilla in small saucepan over medium heat until it registers 140 to 155 degrees, about 5 minutes. Off heat, whisk vigorously to create dense foam on top, about 2 minutes.

3. Remove tea infuser and slowly pour frothed milk over tea, spooning remaining foam over top. Serve immediately.

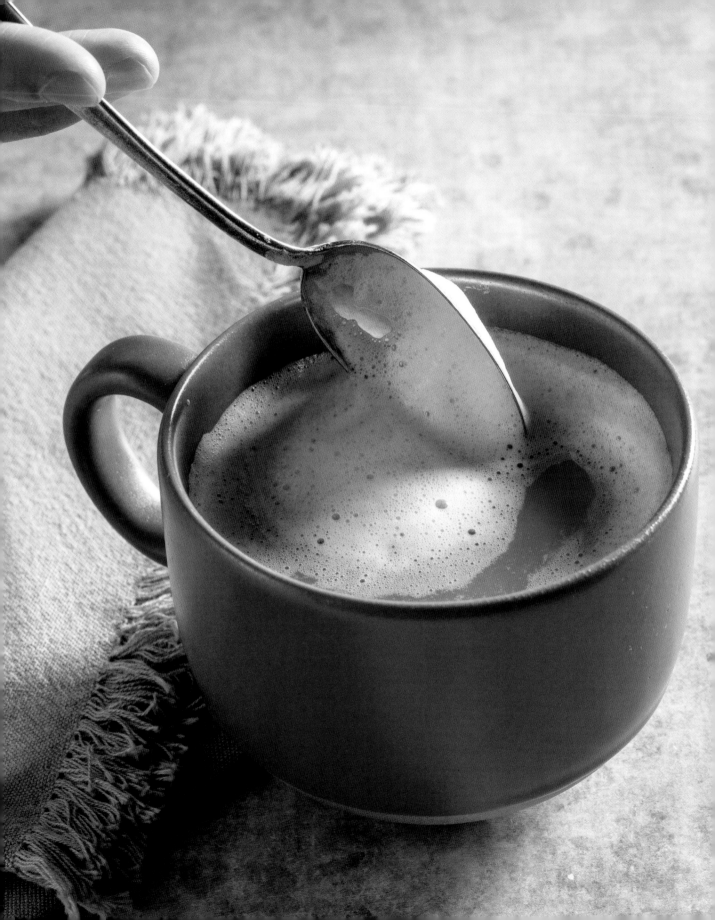

matcha

SERVES 1

1½ teaspoons ceremonial-grade
    matcha powder

1   cup hot water (175 degrees),
    divided

IF YOU DON'T HAVE

ceremonial-grade matcha: Use
premium-grade matcha.

why this combination works: When visiting Ogawa Coffee in Boston, which bases its operations out of Kyoto, Japan, we were given a matcha education and were inspired to learn the process to make it at home. Cultivated in Japan, matcha is a powder made from green tea leaves that are shaded during their growth. This increases the rate of theanine production (an amino acid also found in mushrooms), which gives matcha its characteristic umami taste and determines the quality grade of matcha—the more the plants are shaded, the higher the quality. We found that adding the matcha in two stages, once to make a paste and then the rest to whisk into a froth, resulted in a beverage that had less undissolved sediment. We used 1½ teaspoons of matcha per serving because we found it to have the most complex flavor without being overly bitter, and it resulted in a rich texture. The matcha was strong and produced a thick layer of foam after whisking. Inspired by our visit to Ogawa, we created a matcha latte variation using frothed milk instead of water for subtle sweetness that can turn matcha skeptics into matcha lovers. Avoid culinary-grade matcha. For the latte variation, any type of dairy or nondairy milk will work here; soy milk will yield less foam, so we recommend using an immersion blender.

1. Sift matcha powder into chawan or small soup bowl. Using chasen or small whisk, whisk 2 tablespoons hot water into sifted powder until dissolved. Add another 2 tablespoons hot water and quickly whisk using a zigzag motion until a thick layer of small bubbles form on surface of matcha, about 30 seconds.

2. Stir remaining ¾ cup hot water into matcha. Serve immediately in chawan or teacup.

VARIATION
matcha latte
Omit ¾ cup water in step 2. Heat ¾ cup dairy or plant-based milk in small saucepan over medium heat until it registers 140 to 155 degrees, about 5 minutes. Whisk vigorously to create dense foam on top, about 2 minutes. Slowly pour frothed milk over prepared matcha, spooning remaining foam over top.

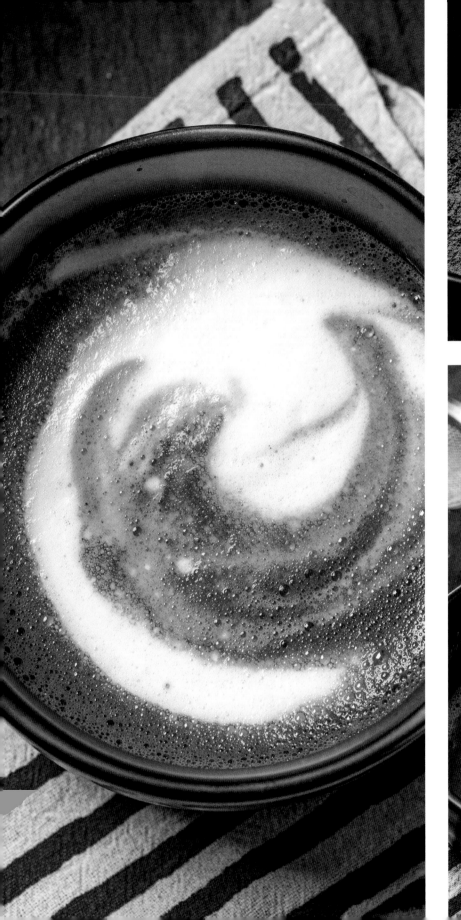
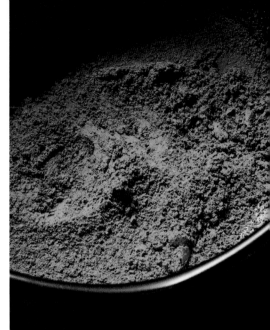
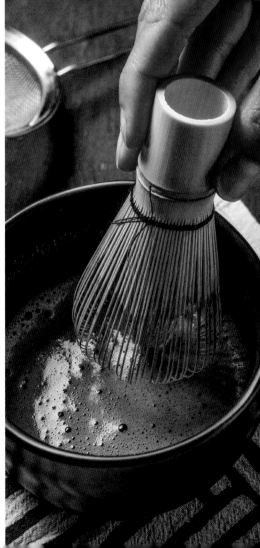

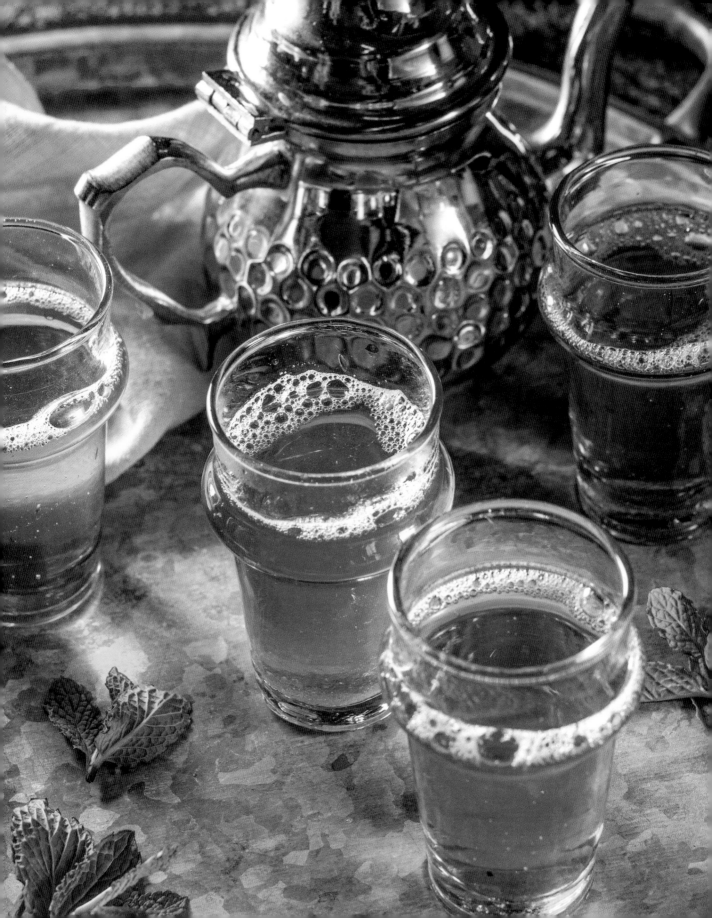

why this combination works: This warm tea is a sweet and refreshing drink that is essential to Moroccan culture and is served to welcome guests. The base of this drink is the gunpowder green tea leaf (named for its rolled, pellet-like shape), which was brought by merchants from China to Morocco in the 1800s. Chef Khalil Aman of Boston generously shared with us how he and his family have been making their mint tea for generations. With only four simple ingredients, preparation is everything. Unlike other green teas, this one is prepared with boiling water. First, the water opens the tea pellets to temper their bitterness. Then, that water is discarded and the washed tea leaves are combined with fresh mint, sugar, and more boiling water, which further softens the astringency of the tea. To serve, the tea is poured from a height to aerate the tea but also to entertain whomever you are sharing the tea with. Gunpowder green tea is also called Lo Chu Ch'a or Zhu Cha. Do not substitute other varieties of tea in this recipe. If your teapot does not have a strainer, transfer the washed tea leaves and mint leaves to a reusable tea infuser or tea sachet before steeping in step 2.

1. Combine ¼ cup boiling water and tea in bowl, then immediately pour off and discard water, reserving tea leaves.

2. Stir remaining 4 cups boiling water, washed tea, mint, and sugar in 6-cup teapot or liquid measuring cup until sugar has dissolved. Cover and let steep for 5 minutes. Working in continuous motion, slowly pour tea into cups while lifting spout of pot away from cups to increase the length and arc of tea stream; return spout of pot to each cup before moving to next cup. Serve immediately with extra mint, if desired.

moroccan mint tea

SERVES 6 TO 8

4¼ **cups boiling water, divided**

4 **teaspoons gunpowder green tea leaves**

½ **cup fresh mint leaves, plus extra for serving**

¼ **cup sugar**

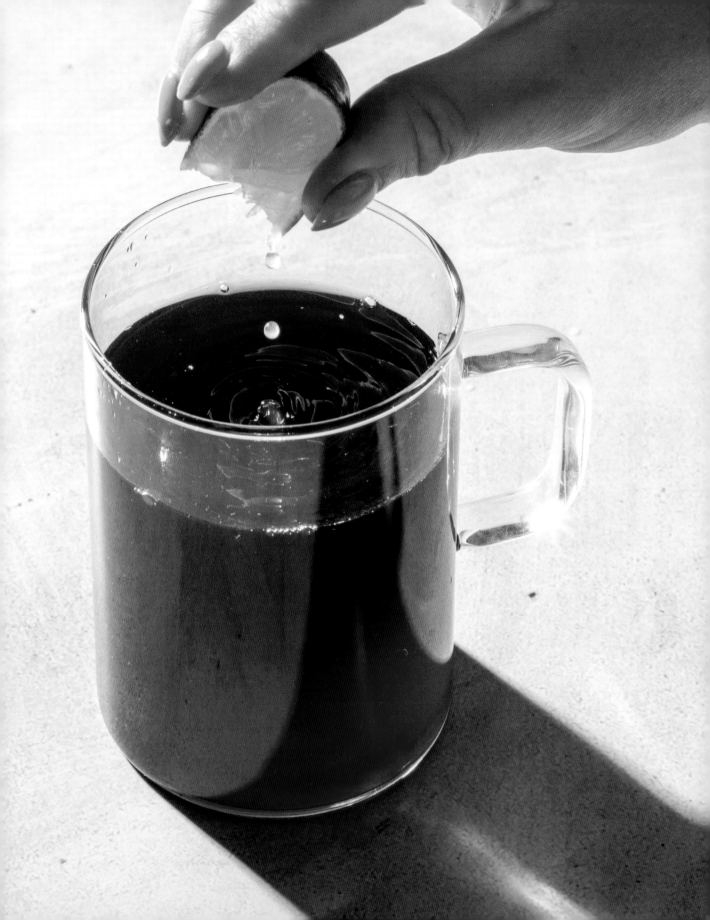

why this combination works: Butterfly pea flower tea, also known as blue tea, is a shockingly colored, caffeine-free, herbal tea. The tea gets its beautiful hue from the petals of a flower native to Asia and has a lightly woodsy taste, similar to green teas. The preparation of this beverage is simple and requires only a straightforward 10-minute steep, so we paid special attention to the balance of flavors to create a drink that tasted as exciting as it looked. Lemongrass provided the tea with a zippy, citrusy flavor that was only slightly mellowed by the boiling water. To further this stimulating flavor profile, fresh ginger brought a pungent and peppery quality that filled our senses with an energizing feel, while a strip of lime zest (and lime wedges for serving) echoed the citrus from the lemongrass with a pleasant and puckering taste. Before slicing lemongrass, trim to bottom 6 inches, then peel and discard tough outer layers. For an accurate measurement of boiling water, bring a kettle of water to a boil and then measure out the desired amount. Butterfly pea flower can be purchased at specialty tea shops, health stores, or online.

Add butterfly pea flower, lemongrass, ginger, and lime zest to tea infuser or tea sachet. Steep tea mixture with boiling water in teacup, covered, for 10 minutes. Remove tea infuser and serve immediately with lime wedges.

butterfly pea flower tea

SERVES 1

- 1 **tablespoon dried butterfly pea flower**
- 1 **teaspoon thinly sliced lemongrass**
- ¼ **teaspoon grated fresh ginger**
- 1 **(3-inch) strip lime zest, plus lime wedges for serving**
- 1 **cup boiling water**

emoliente

SERVES 4

1 **cup roasted barley**

½ **cup flaxseeds**

¼ **cup dried horsetail, crumbled into 1-inch pieces**

1 **stick (2½ inches long by 1 inch wide) cat's claw bark**

2 **quarts water**

3 **tablespoons lemon juice, plus extra for seasoning**

2 **tablespoons honey, plus extra for seasoning**

IF YOU DON'T HAVE

stick cat's claw bark: Use 4 teaspoons chipped or shaved cat's claw bark.

why this combination works: Often sold in the streets of Lima, Peru, emoliente is a warm barley-based beverage made with herb infusions, syrups, and extracts. We wanted to re-create a classic emoliente that would give us the healthful benefits of barley and flaxseeds in a delicious drink. We found several common denominators to emoliente: toasted barley, flaxseeds, horsetail, and cat's claw. Cat's claw is a bitter-tasting, woody vine found in the tropical jungles of South and Central America, while horsetail is a grassy-tasting fern. Toasted barley is chock-full of nutrients and minerals and it gives a nutty flavor when brewed. Flaxseeds gave texture to our beverage and served as a powerhouse of fiber. To meld these flavors together, we introduced lemon juice and honey, which brought a hint of acidity and sweetness that made the final drink taste like warm, sweet-tart lemons with nutty notes, and gave it a thick, soothing texture. Keeping the drink at a simmer for half an hour allowed for proper extraction of the thickening qualities of flaxseeds and for adequate reduction and concentration of flavor. Roasted unhulled barley kernels (sometimes known as toasted barley) is what gives this beverage its distinctive caramel hue and nutty flavor; do not substitute pearl barley. Dried horsetail and cat's claw bark can be purchased at specialty tea shops, health stores, or online.

1. Bring barley, flaxseeds, horsetail, cat's claw, and water to simmer in large saucepan and cook until liquid is reduced by half, 30 to 35 minutes.

2. Strain mixture through fine-mesh strainer into heat-safe bowl, then return to now-empty saucepan. Just before serving, stir in lemon juice and honey. Season with extra to taste. (Emoliente can be refrigerated for up to 3 days; mixture will thicken once chilled but loosen again after reheating. To make a single portion, bring 1 cup emoliente to simmer in small saucepan, then stir in 2 teaspoons lemon juice and 1 teaspoon honey.)

VARIATIONS
emoliente with chamomile
Add 2 tablespoons dried chamomile to saucepan during last 5 minutes of simmering.

emoliente with alfalfa and anise
Add 2 tablespoons dried alfalfa leaves and 1 teaspoon anise seed to saucepan during last 5 minutes of simmering.

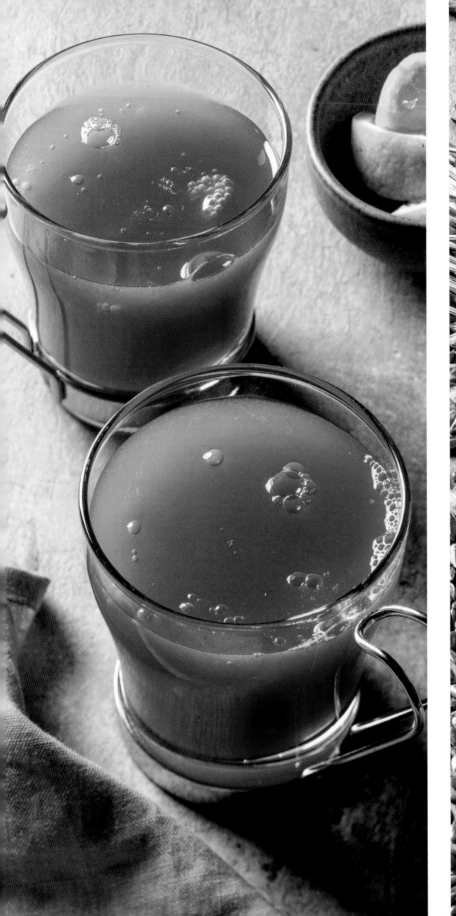
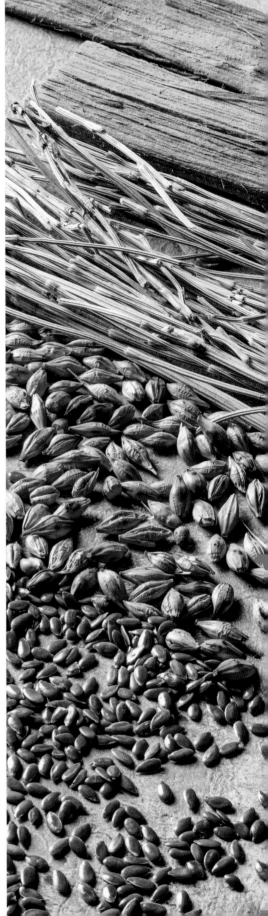

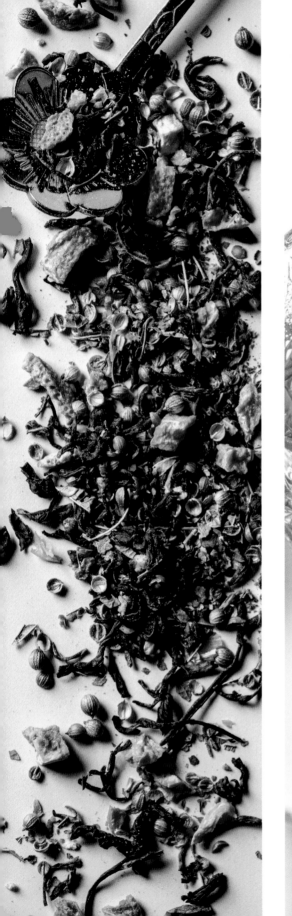
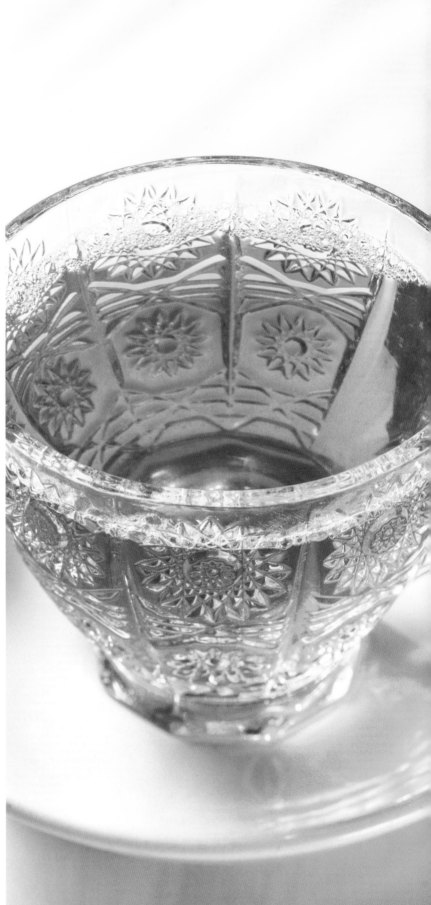

why this combination works: One of the all-time classic pairings is bright and zesty lemon with the earthy, intense tannins of black tea. We wanted to make our own blend at home so we could keep it on hand whenever the craving for a cup strikes—while also controlling the ingredients. We experimented with different forms of this dried blend combination, including lemon peel and lemon balm, but our hands-down favorite was lemon verbena. It added a lemon curd–like richness to the tea because it was both sour and herbal-sweet tasting. To play up the citrus aspect of this tea, dried orange peel brought some floral notes to our blend, while coriander seeds, which already have a citrusy flavor, added savory depth. We used a spice grinder to break up the lemon verbena into manageable and uniform pieces for a well-balanced citrus and black tea flavor. A boldly flavored tea such as Assam is ideal for this recipe; alternatively, use Irish or English breakfast tea. If you have one, a mortar and pestle can be used to crush the spices.

Pulse lemon verbena in spice grinder until coarsely ground and pieces are no larger than ½ inch, about 3 pulses. Add coriander seeds and orange peel and pulse until coarsely ground and pieces of lemon verbena are no larger than ¼ inch, about 4 pulses. Transfer to small bowl and stir in black tea. (Tea blend can be stored in airtight container at room temperature for up to 3 months.)

to make one cup tea: Add 2 teaspoons tea blend to tea infuser or tea sachet. Steep tea mixture with 1 cup boiling water in teacup, covered, for 5 minutes. Remove tea infuser and serve immediately.

citrus burst black tea blend

MAKES 1 CUP DRY BLEND
(ENOUGH FOR 24 SERVINGS)

- ⅔ cup dried lemon verbena
- ⅓ cup coriander seeds
- ⅓ cup dried orange peel
- ⅓ cup black tea leaves

IF YOU DON'T HAVE

coriander seeds: Use fennel seeds.

dried orange peel: Use dried lemon peel.

cacao, cardamom, and rose herbal tea blend

**MAKES 1 CUP
DRY BLEND**

(ENOUGH FOR 16 SERVINGS)

10 green cardamom pods

¾ cup cacao nibs

3 tablespoons dried rose petals

why this combination works: Chocolate and roses don't just make a nice Valentine's Day gift, they also pair nicely in a teacup. Inspired by a black tea blend at a local café, we wanted to make a tisane that combined a rich chocolate flavor with the fragrance of rose petals. Tisanes, often referred to as herbal teas, are infusions made from dried ingredients. We started with dried rose petals, then found our cacao component in the form of whole nibs, which won tasters over—tasting almost of milk chocolate—but the flavor was still a little weaker than we wanted. We tried toasting the nibs, but this made them bitter, so we chose to simply pulse them in a spice grinder to create extra surface area to extract a richer chocolate flavor. With the grinder in use, we took the opportunity to crack some whole cardamom pods, as their aromatic character mimicked that of roses while giving the chocolate a fuller, more spiced expression. If you have one, a mortar and pestle can be used to crush the spices.

Pulse cardamom in spice grinder until coarsely ground, about 10 pulses. Add cacao nibs and pulse until cacao nibs are coarsely ground, about 10 pulses. Transfer to small bowl and stir in rose petals. (Tea blend can be stored in airtight container at room temperature for up to 3 months.)

to make one cup tea: Add 1 tablespoon tea blend to tea infuser or tea sachet. Steep tea mixture with 1 cup boiling water in teacup, covered, for 10 minutes. Remove tea infuser and serve immediately.

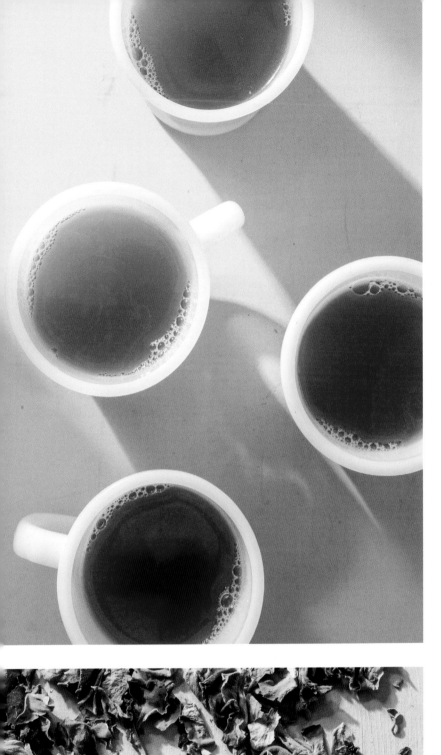
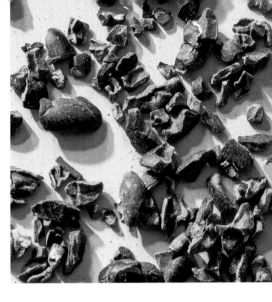
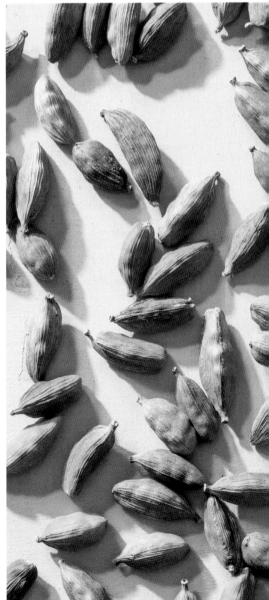
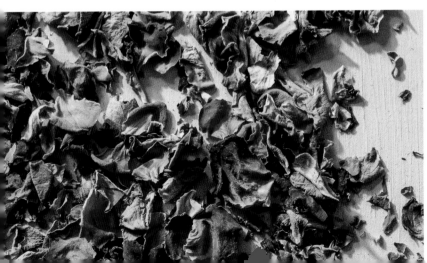

immunitea herbal tea blend

MAKES 1 CUP DRY BLEND

(ENOUGH FOR 16 SERVINGS)

7 **tablespoons dried rose hips**

¼ **cup dried elderberries**

3 **tablespoons dried lemon balm**

3 **tablespoons cut and sifted dried echinacea**

IF YOU DON'T HAVE

cut and sifted dried echinacea:
Use dried echinacea herb or dried echinacea root.

why this combination works: For this blend, we picked herbal components with properties known to boost the immune system, perfect for when you are sick or just want to give your body a fighting chance during the wintertime. Elderberry and rose hips made a fruity-floral base with a tangy quality, similar to hibiscus but with more depth of flavor from the pairing. Elderberries can be effective in reducing the duration of sickness, while rose hips are incredibly high in antioxidants such as vitamin C, which works to prevent illness in the first place. Echinacea, an herbaceous flower, is also full of antioxidants and can reduce the duration of colds and flus. It lent a savory, hay-like taste to the floral blend, and lemon balm provided a light, citrusy flavor with a cooling sensation on the finish to round out the blend. Dried rose hips, lemon balm, and echinacea can be purchased at specialty tea shops, health stores, or online.

Combine all ingredients in a bowl. (Tea blend can be stored in airtight container at room temperature for up to 3 months.)

to make one cup tea: Add 1 tablespoon tea blend to tea infuser or tea sachet. Steep tea mixture with 1 cup boiling water in teacup, covered, for 10 minutes. Remove tea infuser and serve immediately.

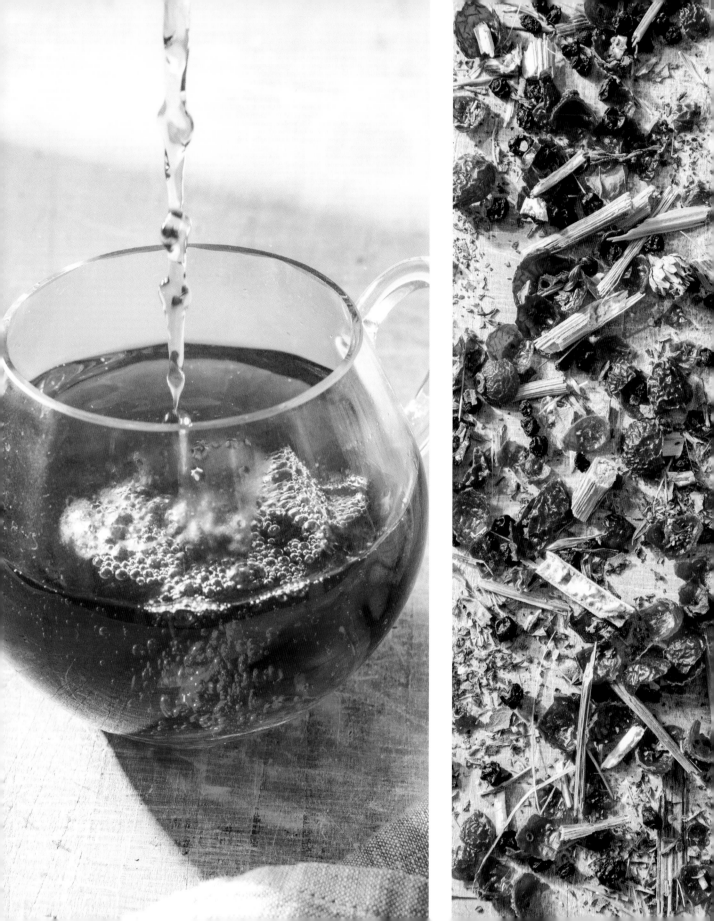

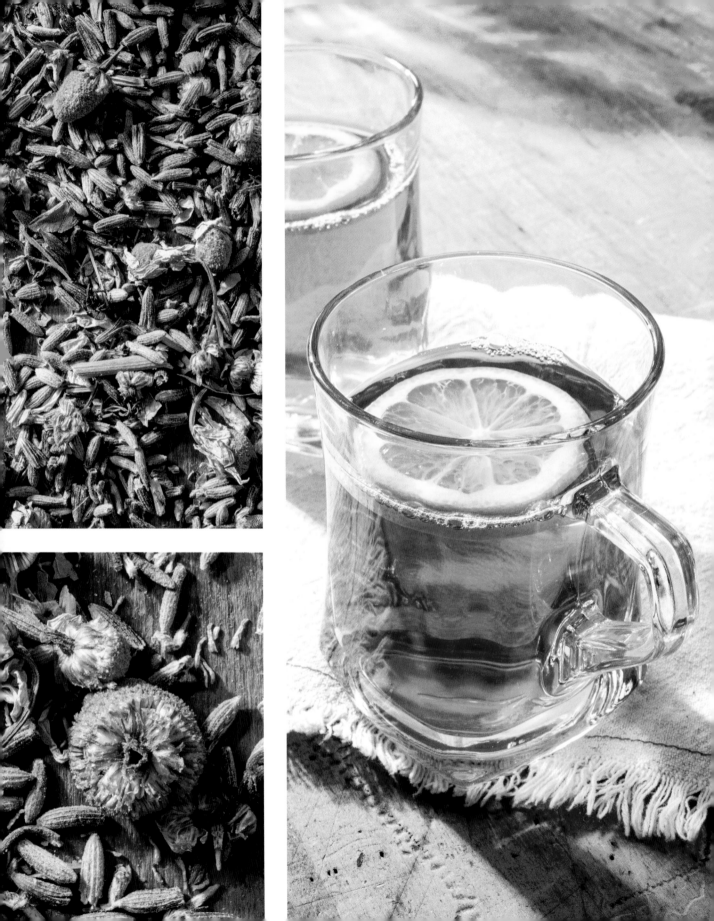

why this combination works: Inspired by well-known relaxing tea blends, we sought to make our own earthy and floral nighttime drink to wind down with at the end of the day. Passionflower, which is grown in South America, has sedative properties that slow down brain activity and promote a feeling of calm. Another potent ingredient in this blend, valerian root, produces mild sedation throughout the body, decreasing anxiety and blood pressure. The valerian root can taste bitter and the passionflower is fairly grassy, so the bulk of our blend was made up of floral ingredients with pleasant aromas to mask those flavors. Dried chamomile and lavender have been used worldwide for their calming properties and sweet botanic taste, so they perfectly completed our roster of cozy ingredients while boosting overall flavor. For an accurate measurement of boiling water, bring a kettle of water to a boil and then measure out the desired amount. Dried passionflower and valerian root can be purchased at specialty tea shops, health stores, or online.

Combine all ingredients in bowl. (Tea blend can be stored in airtight container at room temperature for up to 1 month.)

to make one cup tea: Add 1 tablespoon tea blend to tea infuser or tea sachet. Steep tea mixture with 1 cup boiling water in teacup, covered, for 5 minutes. Remove tea infuser and serve immediately.

cozy and calm herbal tea blend

MAKES 1 CUP DRY BLEND
(ENOUGH FOR 16 SERVINGS)

6 **tablespoons dried chamomile**

5 **tablespoons dried lavender**

2 **tablespoons dried passionflower**

2 **tablespoons dried valerian root**

tummy tea herbal tea blend

MAKES 1 CUP DRY BLEND

(ENOUGH FOR 16 SERVINGS)

⅓ **cup fennel seeds**

¼ **cup dried ginger root**

1 **tablespoon licorice root**

3 **tablespoons dried lemongrass**

3 **tablespoons dried peppermint**

why this combination works: To aid digestion and soothe a sore tummy, this blend of invigorating and beneficial ingredients is also gentle when we need it most. Despite ginger's spicy nature, it is actually an anti-inflammatory that has been known to soothe the intestinal tract and help with nausea. We paired ginger with cooling peppermint, which can relax muscles in the digestive system, and fennel seeds, which have antispasmodic properties to lessen stomach cramps. We enhanced the licoricey flavor of fennel by pairing it with actual licorice root, which added natural sweetness. To get a fuller tasting tea with more body (and no grit), we used a spice grinder to crack the fennel, break up the licorice root, and increase the surface area of the dried ginger root without pulverizing it. Our final ingredient, lemongrass, is a mild diuretic that can reduce uncomfortable bloating; it also gave our blend an additional kick of flavor. The resulting tea is an exploration in opposites because while the flavor is stimulating to the taste buds, the ingredients work to calm and relax the digestive tract. If you have one, a mortar and pestle can be used to crush the spices. Dried ginger root and licorice root can be purchased at specialty tea shops, health stores, or online.

Pulse fennel seeds, ginger, and licorice in spice grinder until coarsely ground, about 10 pulses. Transfer to small bowl and stir in lemongrass and peppermint. (Tea blend can be stored in airtight container at room temperature for up to 3 months.)

to make one cup tea: Add 1 tablespoon tea blend to tea infuser or tea sachet. Steep tea mixture with 1 cup boiling water in teacup, covered, for 10 minutes. Remove tea infuser and serve immediately.

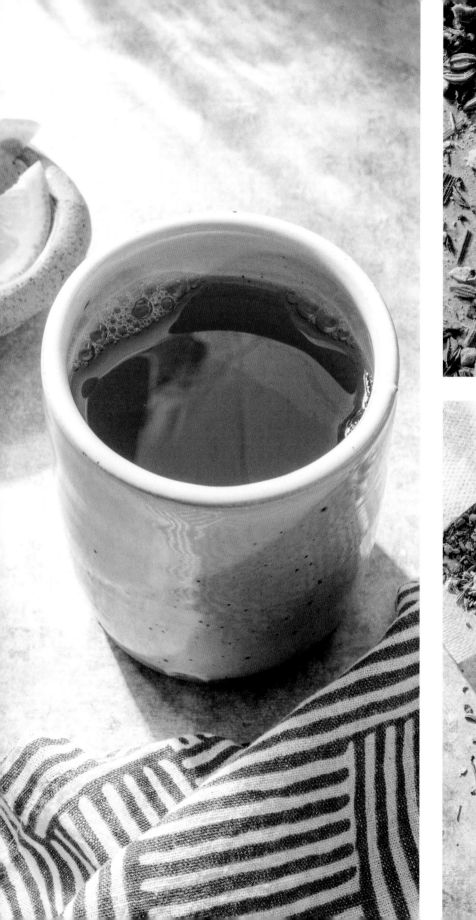
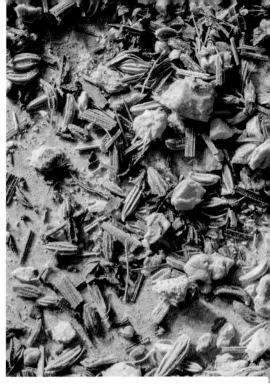
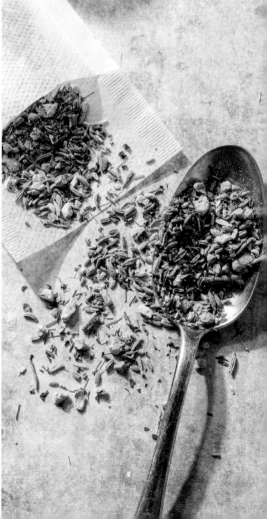

flavored waters

flavored waters 101

Flavored waters are an exciting and convenient way to up your healthful hydration. You may think (and we did too at the start) that you can add a bunch of ingredients to plain old water and expect a tasty result. We quickly realized that we needed to develop a reliable method to add and infuse flavor into water—and make it look good as well. Flavoring your own water means you can make lower-sugar sodas, mocktails, and even our versions of sports drinks and protein shakes that taste great and aren't a compromise. Taste is everything, and adding flavor to water at home means you can have it your way: still or sparkling, fruity or savory, festive enough for guests, and always way better than store-bought.

WHAT TO KNOW

for still water drinks: Instead of simply combining our cut ingredients with water and hoping for the best, we muddle them together for our still water drinks. We create a concentrate by mashing some of the fresh ingredients with a small amount of water. Then we stir that concentrate into 3 cups of water to infuse it with flavor for 30 minutes to 1 hour. Any less time and the flavor is underextracted. After infusing, we strain out the solids from the concentrate so they don't float in the water and impart bitterness or dull the flavors. By stirring in unmuddled produce at the end, we get the benefits of a final pop of fresh flavor and a beautiful garnish.

for sparkling water drinks: To make a bubbly drink that combines a syrup or concentrated mixture with carbonated water, we use a lift method. This technique involves using a spoon to gently lift the components from the bottom of the glass to combine with the seltzer, without deflating all the bubbles. Lifting instead of stirring ensures a well-mixed and fizzy drink.

for spritzers: To flavor seltzer without any added sugar, we use a food processor. Blitzing fresh fruit with additional elements such as extracts or citrus juice creates a flavorful, all-natural concentrate. We then gently stir seltzer into it for uniquely flavored and fresh homemade spritzers (see pages 183–191).

WHAT TO USE

We had an aha moment while testing muddling methods. Given that we were muddling batches for 6 or more, we discovered that we preferred to use a potato masher rather than a traditional drink muddler. While both will work, the potato masher has more surface area so it breaks down the solids more thoroughly and faster. Because it is wide and flat on the bottom, you can apply more pressure over a larger area easily and evenly. Choose whichever one you prefer or have available. When it's time to combine the muddled mixture with more liquid, we find a small strainer to be essential to remove the solids but keep the flavor (see page 161).

To make sparkling drinks, we love the ease of buying and using plain seltzer. Buying individual cans, rather than one large bottle, helps ensure your beverage will be bubbly. You'll also want a large pitcher on hand, as many of our water recipes serve a crowd.

best infusing techniques

FRUIT VARIETY AFFECTS FLAVOR

Different kinds of the same fruit can have a big effect on the flavor, tartness, and sweetness of the final water. Apples and oranges vary in flavor, so experiment to discover the variety you like best.

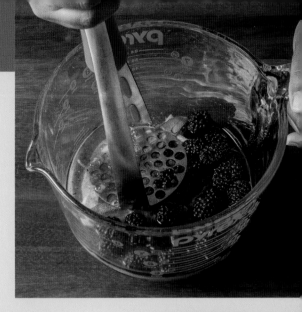

CITRUS IS A GOOD CHOICE

Acidity balanced with sweetness creates complex flavors that work really well in drinks with limited sugar to keep the flavor bold. Thin slices of citrus muddle best to extract not just juice, but more aromatic oils from the zest.

USE SAVORY HERBS

Savory herbs serve to highlight and balance fruit combinations—for instance, using sage with blackberries and grapefruit. Similar to how a pinch of salt draws out flavor, herbs have a similar effect because the contrast creates an interesting new taste fusion.

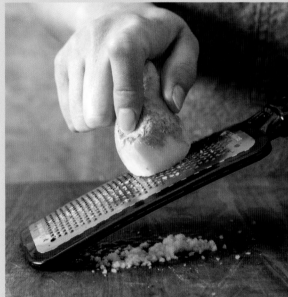

GRATE THE GINGER

Grated ginger is the best way to impart zippy flavor. When cut into rounds, the flavor is dulled because there is less exposed surface area. Grating the ginger releases all its internal flavor compounds, and you can use less grated than sliced ginger.

GENTLY SIMMER SYRUPS

When making flavor-infused simple syrups, bring the ingredients to a gentle simmer. Letting them get too hot will eventually cook out all the flavor you are trying to capture.

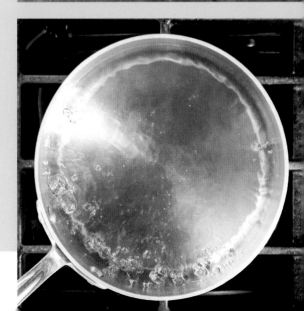

LEARN FROM OUR MISTAKES

As we like to say, during our testing we make the mistakes so you won't have to. First, we learned that infusing our waters for over an hour typically made them bitter, especially when they contain grapefruit. Additionally, we learned that if we didn't strain the muddled mixture, the result was a cloudy and pulpy beverage. Finally, some ingredients just don't infuse well. Lemongrass is a hard and fibrous material that is not extracted well in cold water, no matter how small you cut it. It requires a hot steep rather than a cold infusion, as in Butterfly Pea Flower Tea (page 143).

HOW LONG WILL IT KEEP?

You might think it would be nice to keep a pitcher of cucumber water in the fridge all week, but infused waters really only have a 24-hour shelf life. With all fresh ingredients, infused waters start to turn dull in flavor and lose their vibrancy after more than a day. It is also important to reserve final garnishes on the side to add later. Left in the drink during storage, a fresh garnish will turn mushy and make the water bitter.

STORE-BOUGHT SPARKLING WATER

We love Polar Original Seltzer for its extra-bubbly fizz and crisp, clean flavor. It is nicely carbonated but not so fizzy that it is overwhelming. Overall, it's a neutral, refreshing seltzer that is perfect for mixing up a soda (pages 206–212), creating an alcohol-free cocktail (pages 194–203), or swirling into a spritzer (pages 183–191).

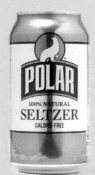

garnishing

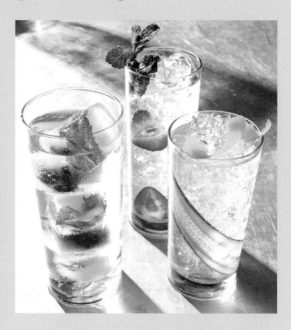

MAKE IT PRETTY

We paid special attention to the visual appeal of our flavored waters. This inspired our muddling method, which calls for reserving some unmuddled produce to be added to the water as a garnish just before serving. Think outside the glass and make garnishes in a variety of ways to add visual interest, whether with simple slices, ribbons, curls, or swizzlers (add ribbons first, then ice). Get creative and don't be afraid to add herb leaves, a decorative sprig, and/or a sprinkle of spice.

NICE ICE

Try adding pieces of fruit, vegetables, citrus, or fresh herbs to your ice cube molds before filling with water for an impressive presentation (see page 209). It's a great way to use up small bits of remaining produce. Keep in mind that any impurities in the water may result in cloudy ice.

water infuser's toolkit

While none of this equipment is essential to water infusing, these items are certainly a help. See Equipment We Use (page 10) for other useful pieces, such as a soda maker.

POTATO MASHER
Muddling is an important technique for properly infusing waters, and we love using a potato masher because of its increased surface area. Our winning potato masher is the **Zyliss Stainless Steel Potato Masher**.

MUDDLER
For a traditional muddler, we like the double-headed **Fletchers' Mill Maple Muddler**. It has a large, smooth head that is easy to grip, even when wet.

LIQUID MEASURING CUPS
Whether used for measuring or as a container to muddle in, 1-cup and 8-cup liquid measuring cups are recommended. Our winning cups are made by **Pyrex**.

SMALL STRAINER
Small strainers sift and strain a variety of ingredients with ease. Both the **Rösle Stainless Steel Fine Mesh Tea Strainer** and the **Küchenprofi Heavy Duty Fine Mesh Stainless Steel 3-Inch Classic Strainer** produce crystal-clear lemon juice, and the weight of their handles and baskets are evenly balanced.

BARSPOON
A long spoon is perfect for gently stirring together a drink and for lifting syrup from the bottom of the glass to mix it in. Our winning barspoon is the **Cocktail Kingdom Teardrop Barspoon**.

PITCHER
When making infused water for a crowd, you need a big sturdy pitcher. If a recipe says it serves 6 to 8, we suggest using a 3- to 4-quart pitcher.

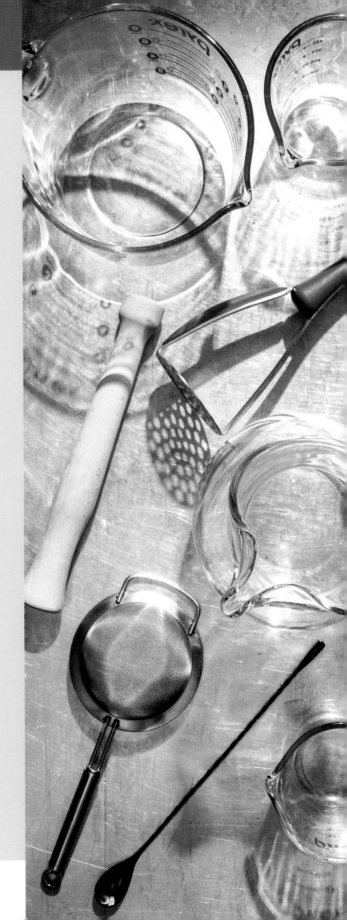

cucumber water

SERVES 6 TO 8

8 **cups water, divided**

12 **ounces cucumber, sliced thin, plus extra for garnish**

why this combination works: We all know that staying hydrated is important, so we turned to infusions to liven up our healthful hydration. During testing, we discovered that the secret to waters with intense flavor and beautiful presentation was dividing the ingredients into muddling items and garnishing items. This allowed us to mash together and extract all the essential flavors during infusing, while leaving extra to float prettily in the glass for our final product. As a result, this water is refreshingly vegetal and clean-tasting. When you want something a little more exciting, our variations offer zippy citrus and an additional flavor component for an easy upgrade. Be sure that all the ingredients are fresh and of good quality. For ideal flavor, enjoy this infused water on the same day of its preparation. Any kind of cucumber will work in this recipe.

1. Combine 1 cup water and three-quarters of the cucumber in 8-cup liquid measuring cup or large bowl. With potato masher or muddler, muddle cucumber until broken down and all juice is expressed, about 30 seconds. Stir in 3 cups water. Cover and refrigerate until flavors meld and mixture is chilled, 30 minutes to 1 hour.

2. Strain infused water into pitcher, pressing on solids to extract as much juice as possible. Discard solids. Stir in remaining 4 cups water and garnish with extra cucumber. (Water can be stored in refrigerator for up to 1 day; garnish with cucumber just before serving.) Serve in ice-filled glasses.

VARIATIONS

cucumber water with lemon and mint
Muddle ½ thinly sliced lemon and ¾ cup fresh mint leaves with cucumber. Garnish with extra thinly sliced lemon and mint leaves.

cucumber water with lime and ginger
Muddle 1 thinly sliced lime and 1 tablespoon grated fresh ginger with cucumber. Garnish with extra thinly sliced lime.

cucumber water with orange and tarragon
Muddle ½ thinly sliced orange and ¾ cup fresh tarragon leaves with cucumber. Garnish with extra thinly sliced orange and tarragon leaves.

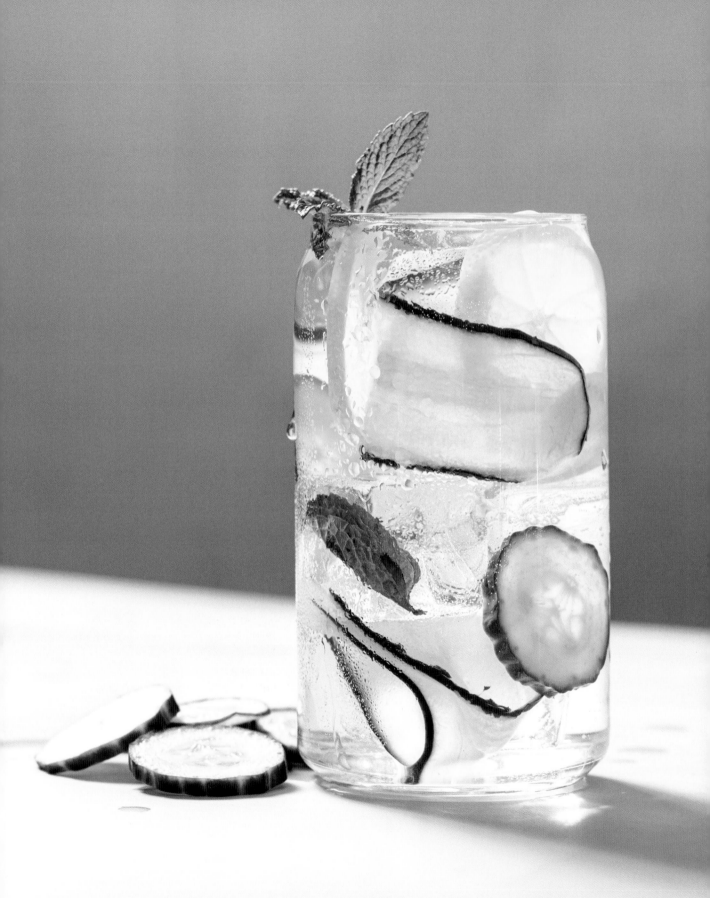

green apple, lemon, and dill water

SERVES 6 TO 8

1 Granny Smith apple, cored and shredded, plus extra for garnish

½ lemon, sliced thin, plus extra for garnish

¼ cup fresh dill, plus extra for garnish

8 cups water, divided

IF YOU DON'T HAVE

Granny Smith apple: Use Fuji, Gala, or Honeycrisp apple.

why this combination works: For a naturally flavored apple water, we experimented with infusing different varieties to achieve the most exciting flavor. We tried Braeburn, Honeycrisp, Fuji, McIntosh, and Golden Delicious apples only to discover that although they all worked just fine, they were very similar—tasty, but generic. When we tested Granny Smiths, however, they stood out as distinctly green and bright, in both color and flavor. Granny Smiths taste almost sour in their intensity, but this quality was lessened once infused, so we emphasized it with a little fresh lemon. Adding dill gave the water an herbal flavor that stood up against the tart apples and lemon while enhancing the fresh taste of this infused water.

1. Combine apple, lemon, dill, and 1 cup water in 8-cup liquid measuring cup or large bowl. With potato masher or muddler, muddle fruit until broken down and all juice is expressed, about 30 seconds. Stir in 3 cups water. Cover and refrigerate until flavors meld and mixture is chilled, 30 minutes to 1 hour.

2. Strain infused water into pitcher, pressing on solids to extract as much juice as possible. Discard solids. Stir in remaining 4 cups water and garnish with extra apple, lemon, and dill. (Water can be stored in refrigerator for up to 1 day; garnish with extra apple, lemon, and dill just before serving.) Serve in ice-filled glasses.

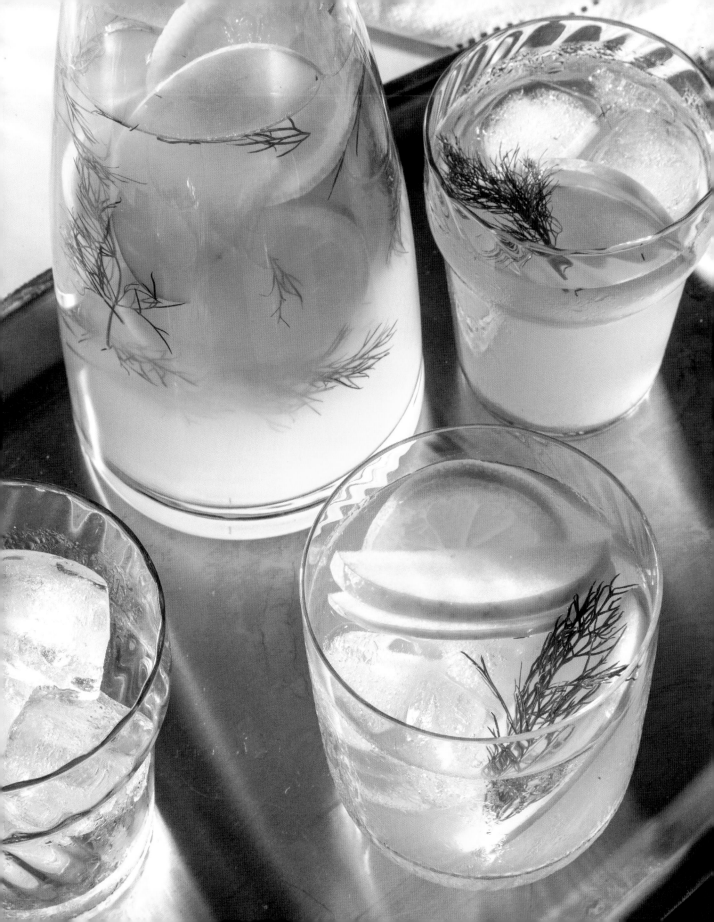

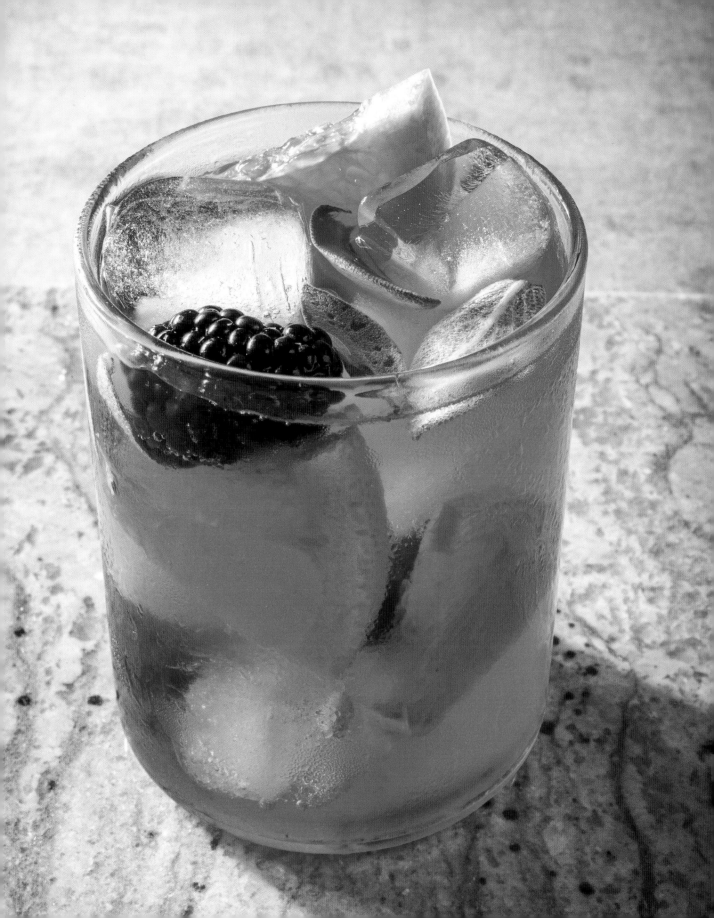

why this combination works: For a citrus- and herb-infused water that used less-traditional ingredients, we turned to grapefruit and sage. Grapefruit gave this water some welcome acidity tinged with bitter notes from the oils present in the peel, which we left on during muddling. Sage offered a complex herbal quality that is both aromatic and grassy. Our final ingredient was blackberries, which provided beautiful color and a sweet flavor to offset the bitter grapefruit, plus they were easy to mash. To allow the herbaceous flavor of this water to hold its own against the strong citrus and berries, we used fresh sage. Together the ingredients played off each other and combined their sweet-tart notes and woodsy herb elements. Be sure to seek out unbruised sage and good-quality ripe blackberries. The grapefruit should not be damaged or bruised. Do not infuse for longer than 1 hour, as the grapefruit steadily takes over the other flavors. For ideal flavor, enjoy this infused water on the same day of its preparation.

1. Combine grapefruit, blackberries, sage, and 1 cup water in 8-cup liquid measuring cup or large bowl. With potato masher or muddler, muddle fruit until broken down and all juice is expressed, about 30 seconds. Stir in 3 cups water. Cover and refrigerate until flavors meld and mixture is chilled, 30 minutes to 1 hour.

2. Strain infused water into pitcher, pressing on solids to extract as much juice as possible. Discard solids. Stir in remaining 4 cups water and garnish with extra grapefruit, blackberries, and sage. (Water can be stored in refrigerator for up to 1 day; garnish with extra grapefruit, blackberries, and sage just before serving.) Serve in ice-filled glasses.

grapefruit, blackberry, and sage water

SERVES 6 TO 8

½ **grapefruit, sliced thin, plus extra for garnish**

1 **cup blackberries, plus extra for garnish**

2 **tablespoons fresh sage leaves, plus extra for garnish**

8 **cups water, divided**

IF YOU DON'T HAVE

blackberries: Use raspberries.

sage: Use 4 thyme sprigs or tarragon.

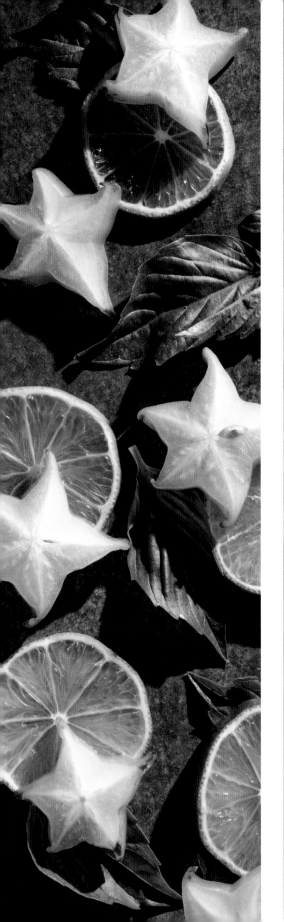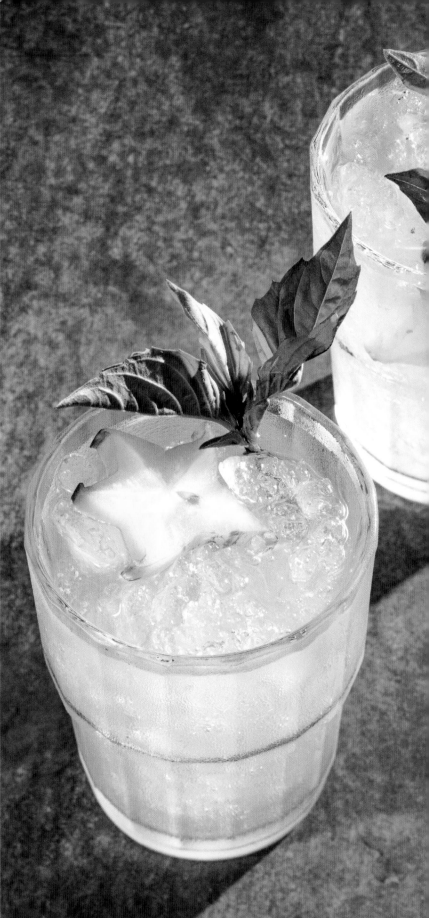

why this combination works: When we began working with a Southeast Asian flavor profile, star fruit became the unexpected star (no pun intended) of this lively infused water. Uniquely shaped and aptly named, star fruit has a sweet-sour honeysuckle flavor that is reminiscent of a kiwi, with similarly textured, juicy flesh. For other complementary flavors, we chose lime juice and Thai basil, which are often found in Southeast Asian drinks. When testing, we experimented with differing amounts of muddled lime and discovered that we enjoyed the high levels of brightness and sour acidity that one whole sliced lime brought to the water. Our herbal element of Thai basil gave the drink a refreshing, licorice-like flavor that combined with the lime and star fruit to taste deliciously invigorating. Star fruit will turn from green to yellow as it ripens; for best results, look for star fruits that are mostly yellow.

1. Combine star fruit, lime, Thai basil, and 1 cup water in 8-cup liquid measuring cup or large bowl. With potato masher or muddler, muddle fruit until broken down and all juices are expressed, about 30 seconds. Stir in 3 cups water. Cover and refrigerate until flavors meld and mixture is chilled, 30 minutes to 1 hour.

2. Strain infused water into pitcher, pressing on solids to extract as much juice as possible. Discard solids. Stir in remaining 4 cups water and garnish with extra star fruit, lime, and basil. (Water can be stored in refrigerator for up to 1 day; garnish with extra star fruit, lime, and basil just before serving.) Serve in ice-filled glasses.

star fruit, lime, and basil water

SERVES 6 TO 8

1½ **star fruits, sliced thin, plus extra for garnish**

1 **lime, sliced thin, plus extra for garnish**

¾ **cup fresh Thai basil leaves, plus extra for garnish**

8 **cups water, divided**

IF YOU DON'T HAVE

Thai basil: Use Italian basil or tarragon.

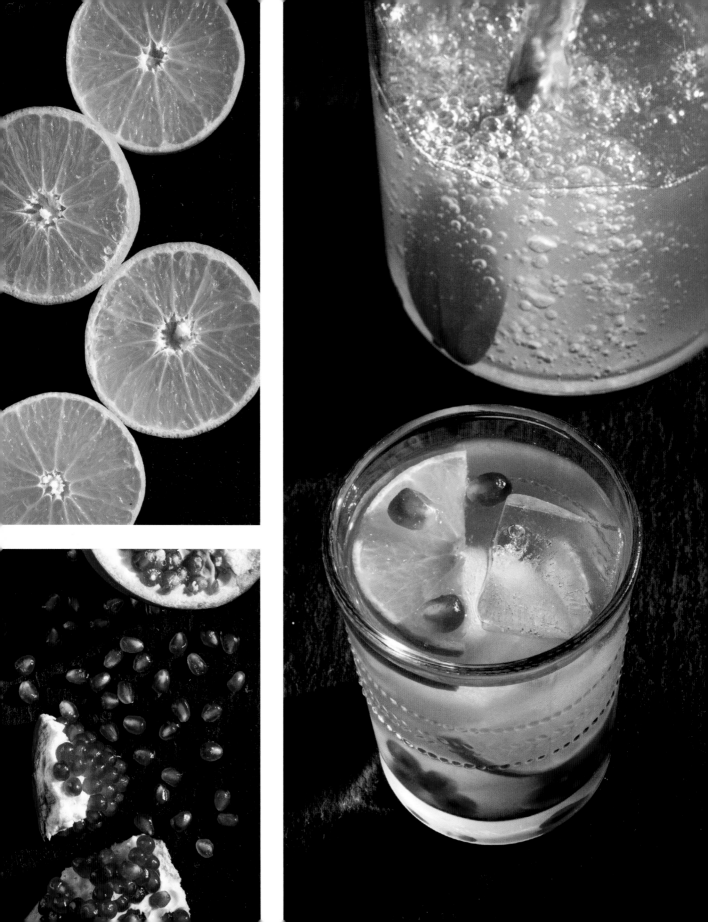

why this combination works: Walking around the grocery store in January in New England and seeing very few brightly colored fruits available inspired us to create this winter-friendly fruit water. While berries looked sad and pale in the dead of winter, the citrus stand was a beacon of bright yellows, oranges, and greens that brought to mind a ray of sunshine. Mandarin oranges had the most inviting color, so they became the base of our drink. What else was in season? Big, beautiful pomegranates. Mandarins have a distinctly juicy, sweet flavor and are lower in acid than other oranges. Pomegranates, on the other hand, are intensely sour and vibrant (in both acidity and color). The addition of ½ cup of seeds livened up the orange, and the bright flavors melded deliciously to create an appealingly tart berryish combo.

1. Combine orange, pomegranate seeds, and 1 cup water in 8-cup liquid measuring cup or large bowl. With potato masher or muddler, muddle fruit until broken down and all juice is expressed, about 30 seconds. Stir in 3 cups water. Cover and refrigerate until flavors meld and mixture is chilled, 30 minutes to 1 hour.

2. Strain infused water into pitcher, pressing on solids to extract as much juice as possible. Discard solids. Stir in remaining 4 cups water and garnish with extra orange and pomegranate seeds. (Water can be stored in refrigerator for up to 1 day; garnish with extra orange and pomegranate seeds just before serving.) Serve in ice-filled glasses.

winter citrus and pomegranate water

SERVES 6 TO 8

1 **mandarin orange, sliced thin, plus extra for garnish**

½ **cup pomegranate seeds, plus extra for garnish**

8 **cups water, divided**

IF YOU DON'T HAVE

mandarin orange: Use blood orange.

pink lemonade

SERVES 6 TO 8

1 **pound strawberries, hulled and halved (2¾ cups)**

1 **lemon, sliced thin, plus 1 cup juice (6 lemons), plus extra slices for garnish**

⅓ **cup honey**

7 **cups water, divided**

why this combination works: Nothing quenches thirst better than a tall, ice-filled glass of the iconic summer staple, pink lemonade. Instead of the store-bought powdered mix that is loaded with sugar, we wanted to re-create the characteristic color and flavor of pink lemonade using a less-processed sweetener. We chose vibrant red ripe strawberries to muddle with lemon slices and naturally produced honey. We used the method we developed for our infused waters here with great success: muddling the strawberries and honey with lemon (peel intact) to extract the oils and punch up the lemon flavor. The muddled mixture was then combined with water and infused before straining out the solids and combining it with freshly squeezed lemon juice and more water. The result is a pink delight, with sweetness provided by the fresh berries and honey and sourness coming from the lemon. Do not substitute bottled lemon juice, as fresh lemons serve as the backdrop for this drink. For ideal flavor, infuse the mixture from step 1 for no more than 1 hour and enjoy this infused water on the same day of its preparation.

1. Combine strawberries, lemon slices, and honey in 8-cup liquid measuring cup or large bowl. With potato masher or muddler, muddle fruit until broken down and all juice is expressed, about 30 seconds. Stir in 4 cups water. Cover and refrigerate until flavors meld and mixture is chilled, 30 minutes to 1 hour.

2. Strain infused water into pitcher, pressing on solids to extract as much juice as possible. Discard solids. Stir in lemon juice and remaining 3 cups water and garnish with extra lemon slices. (Lemonade can be stored in refrigerator for up to 1 day; garnish with extra lemon slices just before serving). Serve in ice-filled glasses.

IF YOU DON'T HAVE

strawberries: Use raspberries.

honey: Use agave nectar.

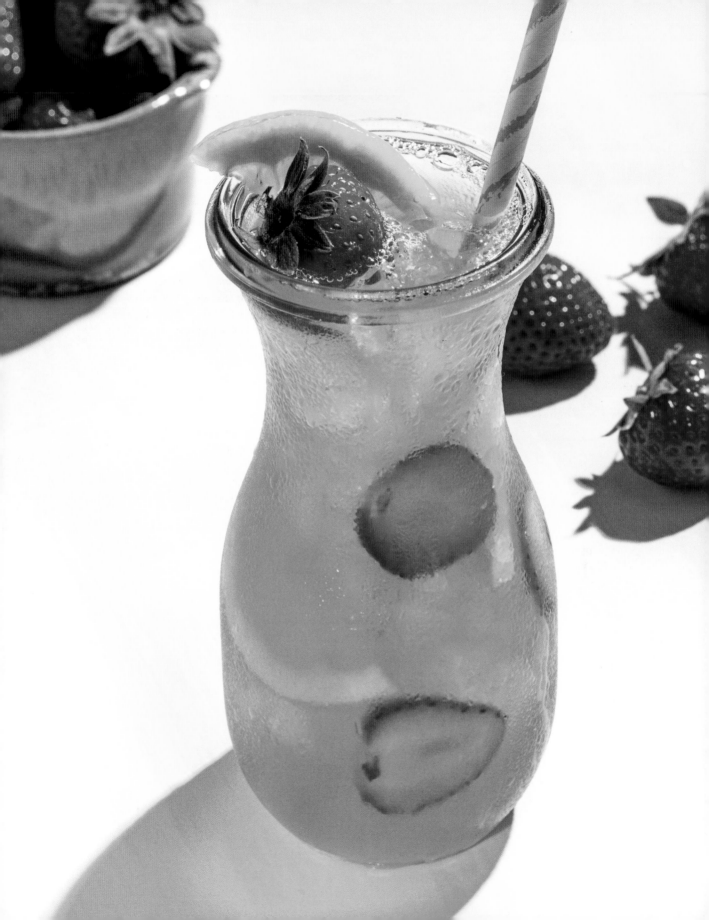

watermelon-lime agua fresca

SERVES 6 TO 8

8 **cups 1-inch seedless watermelon pieces**

2 **cups water**

¼ **cup lime juice (2 limes)**

1–2 **tablespoons agave nectar**

¼ **teaspoon table salt**

Fresh mint leaves

why this combination works: Agua fresca, or "fresh water," is a refreshing Mexican fruit drink. The phrase also covers a variety of blended beverages made from fruits, grains, seeds, or flowers with sugar and water. To make a version with one of summer's favorite fruits—watermelon—we whizzed chunks of the melon with water in a blender and strained out the pulp before accenting the mixture with lime juice for tartness, agave nectar for sweetness, and a pinch of salt to bring out both those flavors. Agave nectar is extracted as juice from agave plants before being heated to reduce the liquid and concentrate its sweet flavor. While similar to honey, it has a more neutral flavor that blends seamlessly into our subtly sweet watermelon and lime drink. Because watermelons vary in sweetness, we started by tasting our watermelon to determine how much agave nectar to incorporate into the agua fresca. Adjust the amounts of lime juice and sweetener to your taste.

Working in 2 batches, process watermelon and water in blender until smooth, about 30 seconds. Strain mixture through fine-mesh strainer into pitcher; discard solids. Stir in lime juice, agave, and salt until agave and salt have dissolved. Serve in ice-filled glasses, garnished with mint. (Agua fresca can be refrigerated for up to 5 days; stir to recombine before serving.)

IF YOU DON'T HAVE

agave nectar: Use honey.

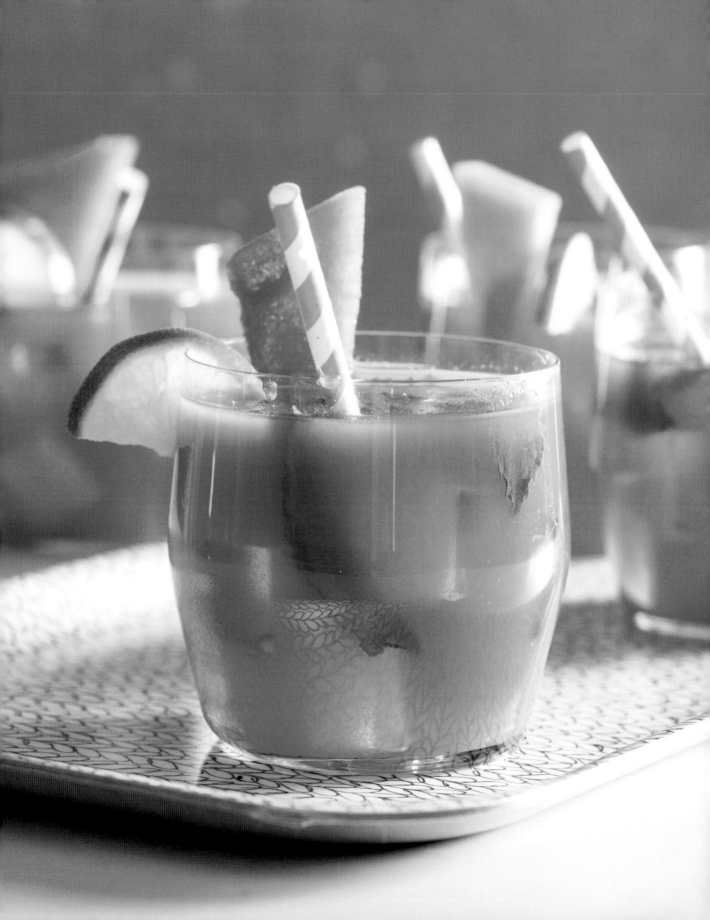

honeydew-lemon agua fresca

SERVES 6 TO 8

8 **cups 1-inch honeydew pieces**

2 **cups water**

¼ **cup lemon juice (2 lemons)**

1–2 **tablespoons agave nectar**

¼ **teaspoon table salt**

Fresh basil leaves (optional)

why this combination works: This honeydew melon and lemon agua fresca is a great way to switch up your hydration game or provide your brunch guests with an exciting alcoholic-free beverage. To keep this drink only mildly sweet, we derived sweetness from the melon itself and a bit of added agave nectar. Honeydew melon has a juicy but mild flavor, so we enlivened it with punchy lemon juice. Using only ¼ cup allowed us to make the overall drink bolder tasting, while letting the citrus mellow into the background and not turn the drink sour. This beverage keeps for days, so if you make it ahead, you have a better-than-bottled beverage to grab on your way out of the house all week. Because honeydew melons vary in sweetness, we started by tasting our honeydew to determine how much agave nectar to incorporate into the agua fresca. Adjust the amounts of lemon juice and sweetener to your taste.

Working in 2 batches, process honeydew and water in blender until smooth, about 30 seconds. Strain mixture through fine-mesh strainer into pitcher; discard solids. Stir in lemon juice, agave, and salt. Serve in ice-filled glasses, garnished with basil, if using. (Agua fresca can be refrigerated for up to 5 days; stir to recombine before serving.)

IF YOU DON'T HAVE

honeydew: Use cantaloupe.

agave nectar: Use honey.

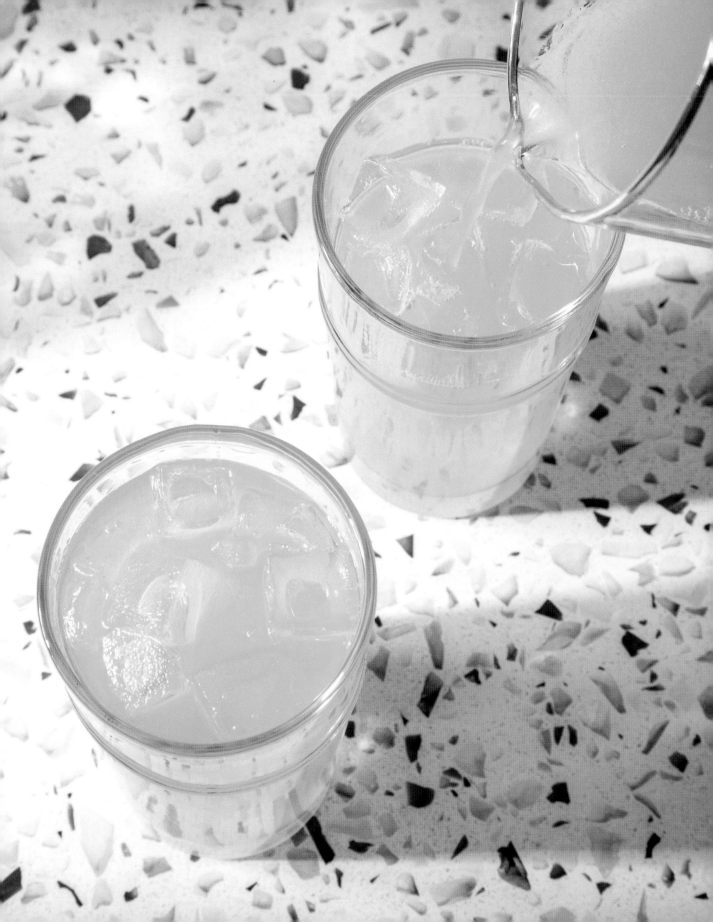

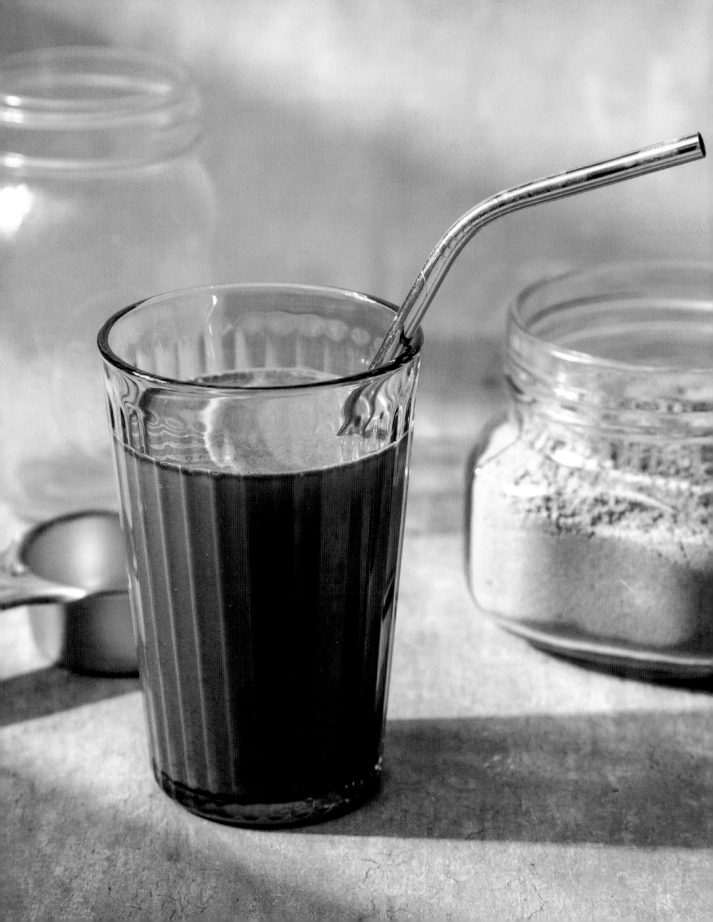

why this combination works: Using flavored protein powder puts your health in your own hands by giving you control over your protein source. And making your own powdered mix allows you to shake up only what you want to drink that day, so nothing goes to waste. We balanced readily available unflavored whey protein isolate with a touch of sugar, spice, and chocolate for a superlative shake. For our primary recipe, we chose crowd-pleasing chocolate in the form of unsweetened cocoa powder so we could get that chocolaty flavor but still keep sugar amounts in check. To switch up the flavor profile and add a bit of caffeine for additional pre-workout power, we created two variations with warm spices: one with espresso powder and another with matcha powder. Do not substitute whey protein concentrate for the whey protein isolate powder. This recipe can easily be doubled.

1. for the dry mix: Whisk whey protein powder, cocoa, sugar, and cinnamon, if using, together in bowl; transfer to storage container with tight-fitting lid.

2. for each shake: Combine 1 cup milk and rounded ¼ cup dry mix in 2- to 4-cup beverage container with tight-fitting lid. Seal container and shake vigorously until protein mix has fully dissolved, about 30 seconds. Serve.

VARIATIONS
matcha-cardamom protein shake
Substitute matcha powder for cocoa powder and ground cardamom for cinnamon.

spiced coffee protein shake
Substitute espresso powder for cocoa powder and 2 teaspoons five-spice powder for cinnamon.

chocolate protein shake

MAKES 2¼ CUPS POWDERED PROTEIN MIX
(ENOUGH FOR 8 SHAKES)

DRY MIX

2 cups (6 ounces) unflavored whey protein isolate powder

¼ cup (¾ ounce) unsweetened cocoa powder

2 tablespoons sugar

2½ teaspoons ground cinnamon (optional)

SHAKE

Dairy or plant-based milk

IF YOU DON'T HAVE

milk: Use water.

strawberry electrolyte refresher

MAKES ⅔ CUP DRY MIX
(ENOUGH FOR 8 REFRESHERS)

DRY MIX

- ½ **cup (½ ounce) freeze-dried strawberries**
- ½ **cup sugar**
- 1 **teaspoon citric acid**
- ½ **teaspoon table salt**
- ½ **teaspoon dried mint (optional)**

REFRESHER

Water

IF YOU DON'T HAVE

strawberries: Use freeze-dried blueberries, mango, pineapple, raspberries, or tart cherries.

why this combination works: For sports drink lovers, this surprisingly easy homemade powdered mix can be rehydrated with water for any workout or when you need extra hydration on a hot day. Salt, carbohydrates, and water are the essential components of an exercise drink because sodium and chloride are the electrolytes lost when sweating, carbohydrates (from sugar) provide energy, and water hydrates us. For a ready-to-go combo that we could simply mix with water, we turned to freeze-dried fruit. Blitzed up in the blender, they added bursts of fruity flavor and fun attractive colors (without any of the artificial dyes and flavors found in commercial sports drinks). To balance out the drink's sweetness, we used citric acid, which gave just the right amount of acidity but in powdered form. Adding a bit of dried herbs or spices to the mix made them feel personalized while still refreshing and thirst quenching. This great-tasting and hydrating refresher can be ready in 15 minutes, with enough extra mix to make 7 more drinks. You can purchase food-grade citric acid online or in grocery stores that sell canning supplies. You can use a spice grinder if you don't have a blender.

1. for the dry mix: Process strawberries, sugar, citric acid, salt, and mint, if using, in blender until finely ground, about 30 seconds, scraping down sides of blender jar as needed. Using fine-mesh strainer, sift mixture into large bowl; discard any seeds and remaining fruit pieces. Transfer to storage container with tight-fitting lid.

2. for each refresher: Combine 1 cup water and 1 rounded tablespoon dry mix in 2- to 4-cup beverage container with tight-fitting lid. Seal container and shake vigorously until refresher mix is fully combined (fruit powder will not dissolve), about 30 seconds. Serve.

VARIATIONS

blueberry-cinnamon electrolyte refresher
Substitute freeze-dried blueberries for strawberries and ¼ teaspoon ground cinnamon for mint.

tart cherry–fennel electrolyte refresher
Substitute freeze-dried tart cherries for strawberries and ¼ teaspoon ground fennel seeds for mint.

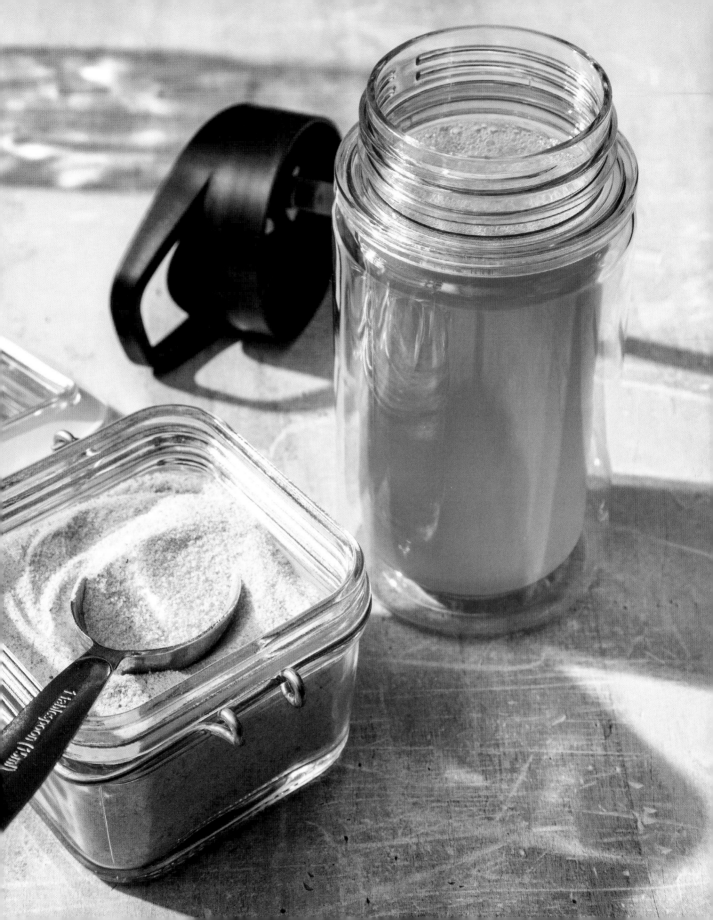

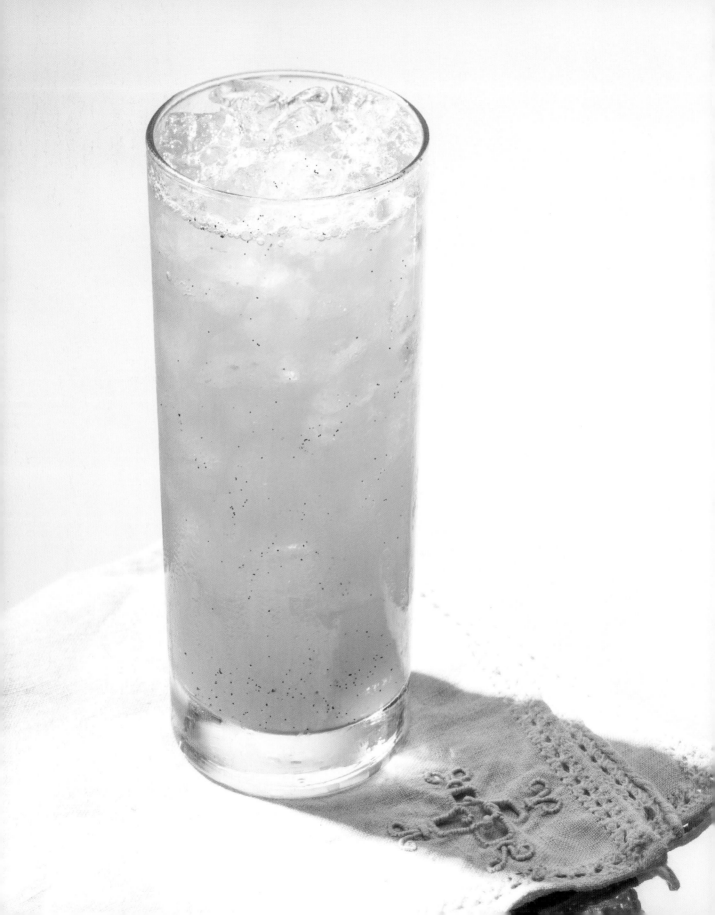

why this combination works: For a sugar-free drink inspired by cream soda, we processed vanilla bean with ripened pears and combined it with bubbly seltzer. We opted to use vanilla bean instead of vanilla extract because while the latter worked in this recipe and is traditionally beneficial in baking, it tasted slightly of alcohol. For enhanced body and added complexity to complement the vanilla flavor, we used pears. The pears tasted vaguely of warm spices and became thick and velvety in the food processor, which added a nice texture to our final drink when the seltzer was stirred in. Be sure that the pear is perfectly ripe for easy prep and a delicious final product. The puree will hold well in the fridge for up to 1 day. It may get slightly darker as the day progresses.

1. Cut vanilla bean in half lengthwise. Using tip of paring knife, scrape out seeds; discard empty pod. Process pears and vanilla seeds in food processor until smooth, scraping down sides of bowl as needed, about 90 seconds. Strain mixture through fine-mesh strainer into pitcher. (Puree can also be stored in airtight container in refrigerator for up to 2 days; transfer puree to pitcher before proceeding.)

2. Just before serving, gently stir seltzer into puree until combined. Pour into ice-filled glasses. (You can also make a single portion by combining ¼ cup puree and ¾ cup seltzer in glass before adding ice.)

pear and vanilla spritzer

SERVES 4 ·

½ **vanilla bean**

2 **Bosc pears, peeled, halved, and cored**

3 **cups seltzer, chilled**

IF YOU DON'T HAVE

vanilla bean: Use ¼ teaspoon vanilla extract.

Bosc pear: Use Anjou or Bartlett pear.

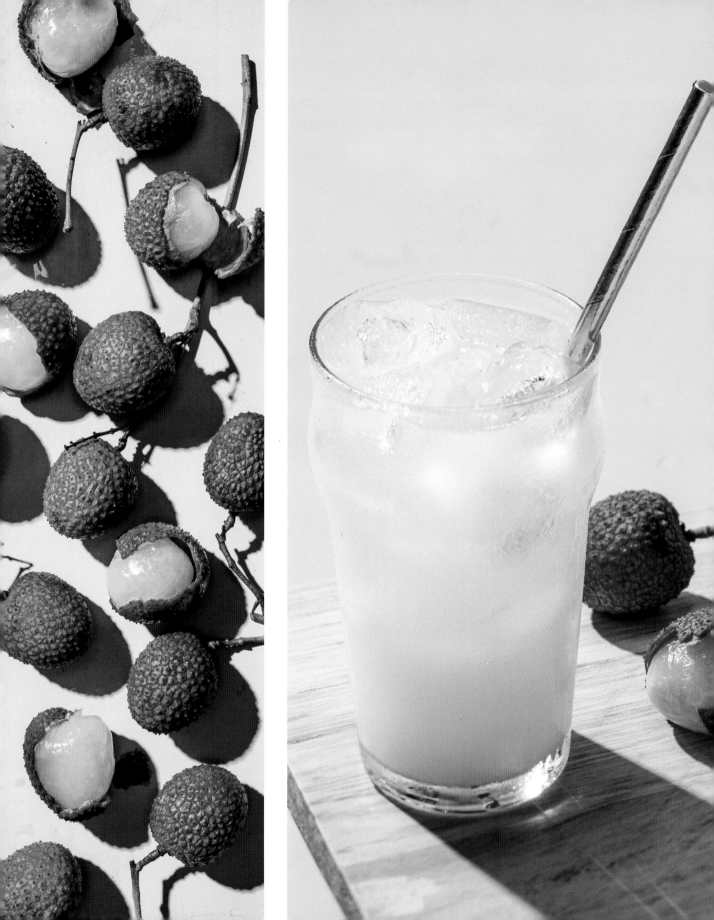

why this combinations works: While exploring unique fruits with elevated flavor, we decided to create a lychee puree that we could mix into seltzer. Lychee is a Southeast Asian berry that is small and easy to peel; it tastes like strawberry crossed with watermelon. We wanted to play up the naturally present floral notes of lychee and found that the convenience and delicate flavor of orange blossom water both complemented and heightened the lychee flavor. Initially, we experimented with rose water and although we liked it, we favored the more delicate flavor of orange blossom water. To prep fresh lychees, be sure to remove the skin and pit. Try to capture any juices that may accumulate on your cutting board. Orange blossom water can be found in the Middle Eastern section of most grocery stores. If fresh lychees are not available, canned lychees can be used instead; make sure to drain and rinse them. Fresh lychees make a rosy pink puree and canned lychees a milky white color.

1. Process lychees and orange blossom water in food processor until smooth, scraping down sides of bowl as needed, about 1 minute. Strain mixture through fine-mesh strainer into pitcher. (Puree can also be stored in airtight container in refrigerator for up to 2 days; transfer puree to pitcher before proceeding.)

2. Just before serving, gently stir seltzer into puree until combined. Pour into ice-filled glasses. (You can also make a single portion by combining ¼ cup puree and ¾ cup seltzer in glass before adding ice.)

lychee and orange blossom spritzer

SERVES 4

1¼ **pounds fresh lychees, peeled and pitted**

½ **teaspoon orange blossom water**

3 **cups seltzer, chilled**

IF YOU DON'T HAVE

fresh lychees: Use canned peeled and pitted lychees.

orange blossom water: Use rose water.

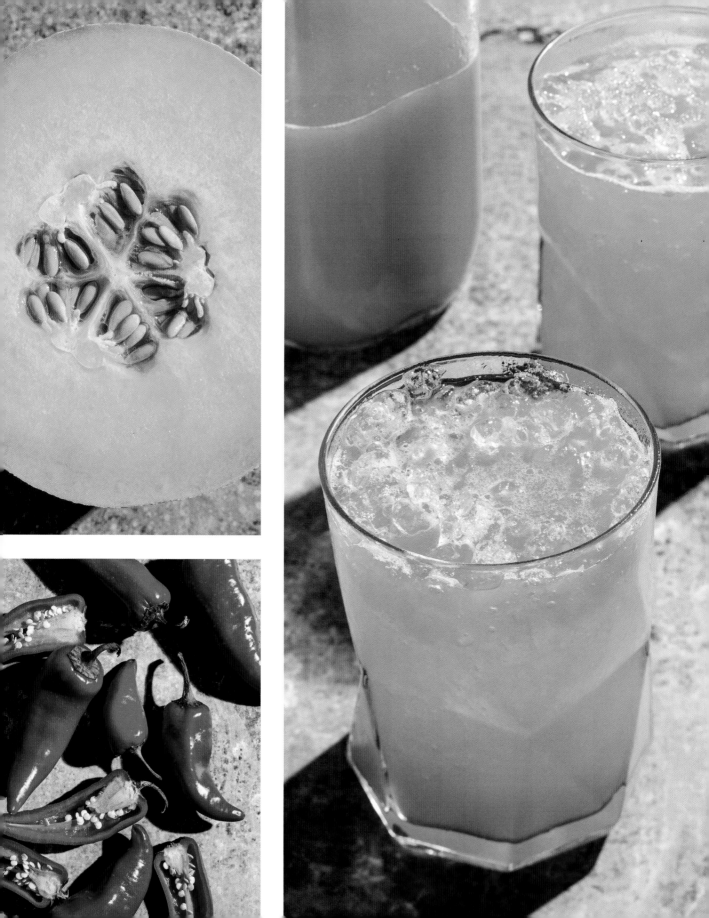

why this combination works: We love the delicately sweet taste of cantaloupe and knew that we wanted to kick it up a notch for a stimulating spritzer. When testing powerful ingredient pairings, we explored mint and melon, which made for a nice flavor combination, but ultimately the pureed mint turned brown and unappetizing looking. Spice and fruit are a proven twosome, so we began to explore Aleppo pepper, cayenne, and Fresno chiles. In the end, we preferred the subtle heat and fresh spiciness of the Fresno. When processed, the cantaloupe created a frothy and colorful puree and the chile deepened the color to a rich orange. When trying different levels of spice, we landed on ½ chile (seeded) for a result that was pleasantly spicy but not painful. Straining the blend before stirring it into seltzer worked to filter out the bits of pepper skin for a smooth drink.

1. Process cantaloupe and chile in food processor until smooth, scraping down sides of bowl as needed, about 1 minute. Strain mixture through fine-mesh strainer into pitcher. (Puree can also be stored in airtight container in refrigerator for up to 2 days; transfer puree to pitcher before proceeding.)

2. Just before serving, gently stir seltzer into puree until combined. Pour into ice-filled glasses. (You can also make a single portion by combining ¼ cup puree and ¾ cup seltzer in glass before adding ice.)

cantaloupe and fresno chile spritzer

SERVES 4

2 **cups 1-inch cantaloupe pieces**

½ **Fresno chile, stemmed, seeded, and chopped**

3 **cups seltzer, chilled**

IF YOU DON'T HAVE

cantaloupe: Use honeydew.

Fresno chile: Use jalapeño.

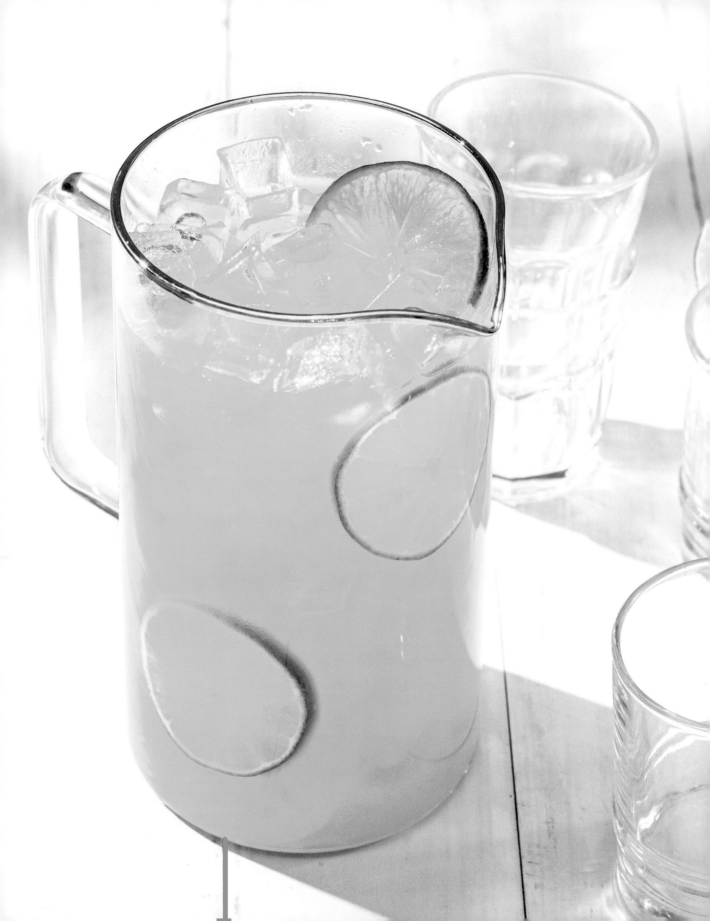

why this combination works: Fresh mango was essential to this spritzer because it is one of only two ingredients; we found that without other flavors to stand behind or meld with in this drink, frozen mango was not assertive enough. While frozen mango is available year-round and is welcome in smoothies, this beverage needed the fresh and juicy flesh of a ripe mango. For a tropical pairing, we processed the fresh mango with lime juice and some intense-tasting zest to add strong lime aroma and much-needed acidity to balance out the sweet fruit. When the mango was broken down in the food processor, it created a beautifully thick puree. Straining this blend was essential to filter out the fruit pulp and the lime zest, which imparted nice flavor but can taste bitter when ingested straight. In addition to plain seltzer, this pureed combination pairs nicely with coconut water, which adds a little body and mild sweetness to the drink.

1. Process mangos and lime zest and juice in food processor until smooth, scraping down sides of bowl as needed, about 1 minute. Strain mixture through fine-mesh strainer into pitcher. (Puree can also be stored in airtight container in refrigerator for up to 2 days; transfer puree to pitcher before proceeding.)

2. Just before serving, gently stir seltzer into puree until combined. Pour into ice-filled glasses. (You can also make a single portion by combining ¼ cup puree and ¾ cup seltzer in glass before adding ice.)

mango and lime spritzer

SERVES 4

- **2 mangos, peeled, pitted, and coarsely chopped**

- **½ teaspoon grated lime zest plus 1 tablespoon juice**

- **3 cups seltzer, chilled**

IF YOU DON'T HAVE

lime: Use lemon or orange.

seltzer: Use coconut water.

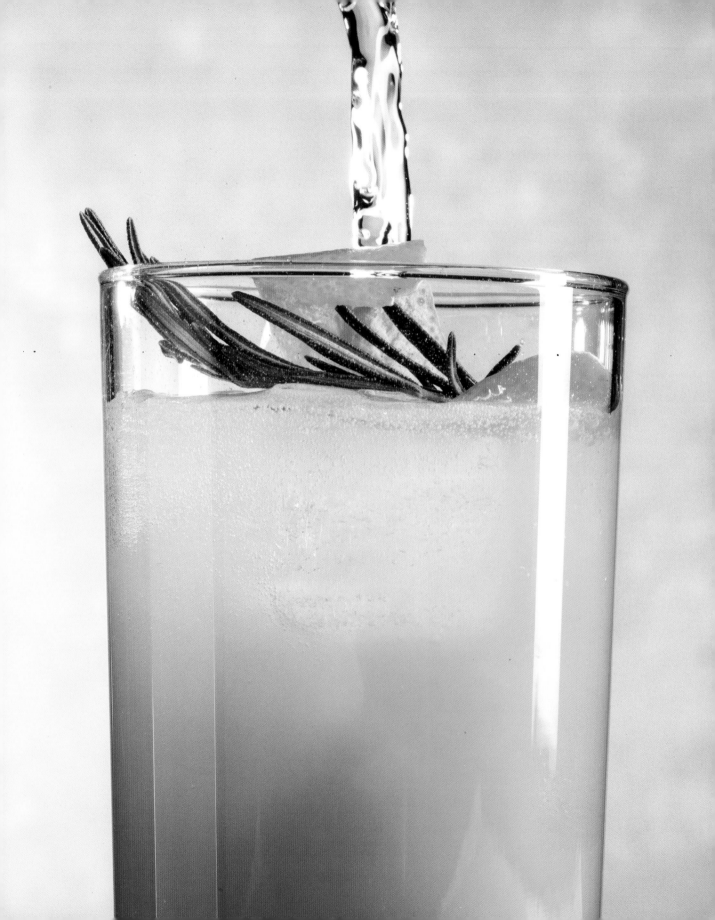

why this combination works: With its citrus and herbal flavors, this simple but sophisticated and not-too-sweet alcoholic-free cocktail is perfect for brightening up your winter holiday table. The three ingredients—freshly squeezed grapefruit juice, seltzer, and rosemary simple syrup—add up to far more than just the sum of their parts. Our preferred method of getting herbal flavors into our drinks is via a flavored syrup (because it disperses so evenly), so rather than muddle in fresh rosemary, we employed our herb simple syrup. The syrup's piney flavor tempered the grapefruit's tartness and gave the drink intriguing savory notes. And because the herb syrup contains some sugar, the intense rosemary and grapefruit flavors were softened. We prefer to use fresh juice for this spritzer (feel free to use yellow, pink, or red grapefruit, as you prefer); however, you can substitute unsweetened store-bought juice. Garnish the spritzers with a rosemary sprig in addition to the grapefruit twist, if you like.

Fill chilled glass halfway with ice. Add grapefruit juice and rosemary syrup and stir to combine. Add seltzer and, using spoon, gently lift juice mixture from bottom of glass to top to combine. Top with additional ice and garnish with grapefruit zest and rosemary sprig, if using. Serve.

grapefruit-rosemary spritzer

SERVES 1

- ½ **cup grapefruit juice plus 1 strip zest, for garnish**
- 1 **tablespoon Herb Syrup with rosemary (page 206)**
- ½ **cup seltzer, chilled**
- **Rosemary sprig, for garnish (optional)**

IF YOU DON'T HAVE

herb syrup with rosemary: Use herb syrup with thyme or sage (page 206).

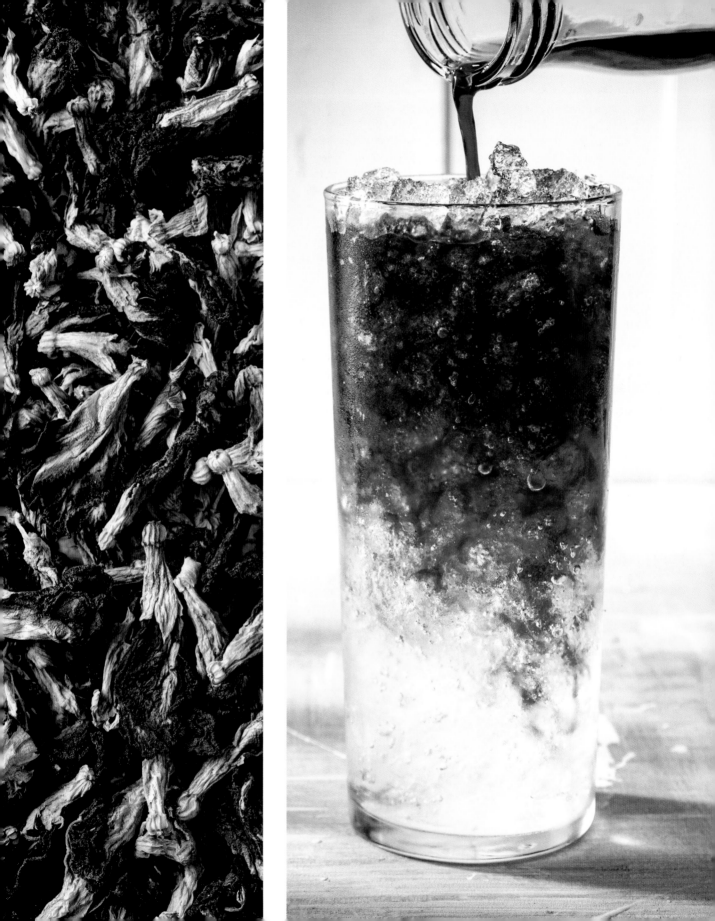

why this combination works: In Thailand and Vietnam, butterfly pea flower tea is a popular drink. While we love it hot (page 143), we wanted to make a visually arresting, super-fun spritzer for the warmer months. Using what we learned in our tea chapter, we tried making this drink with our regular tea, but the flavor was too muted once chilled. To combat this, we doubled the concentration and used our iced tea method (instead of our hot one) so we could draw out more of the delicate floral flavors of the tea. The color starts blue in a neutral or basic environment and turns progressively red as more acid is introduced. A little lime juice added directly to the glass with seltzer turned the drink a beautiful purple. To get the layering effect, we filled the bottom of the glass with honey, seltzer, and lime, then poured the blue tea onto the ice so the distinct layers were maintained. Before mincing lemongrass, trim to bottom 6 inches, then peel and discard tough outer layers. For an accurate measurement of boiling water, bring a kettle of water to a boil and then measure out the desired amount. Butterfly pea flower can be purchased at specialty tea shops, health stores, or online.

1. Place butterfly pea flower, lemongrass, and ginger in medium bowl. Add boiling water and let steep for 10 minutes. Add ice water and steep for 1 hour. Strain through fine-mesh strainer into container. Stir in honey until dissolved. Refrigerate until chilled, at least 1 hour or up to 3 days.

2. Fill 2 chilled glasses with ice. Add ½ cup seltzer and ½ teaspoon lime juice to each glass and stir to combine. Gently pour in ½ cup prepared butterfly pea flower tea. Top with additional ice and serve.

butterfly pea flower spritzer

SERVES 2

- **2 tablespoons dried butterfly pea flower**
- **2 teaspoons minced lemongrass**
- **½ teaspoon grated fresh ginger**
- **¾ cup boiling water**
- **¼ cup ice water**
- **1 teaspoon honey**
- **1 cup seltzer, divided**
- **1 teaspoon lime juice, divided**

IF YOU DON'T HAVE

honey: Use agave nectar.

lime juice: Use lemon juice.

bubbly sage cider

SERVES 1

¼ cup apple cider

1 tablespoon Herb Syrup with sage (page 206)

½ teaspoon apple cider vinegar

¾ cup seltzer, chilled

Apple slices, for garnish (optional)

Fresh sage leaves, for garnish (optional)

IF YOU DON'T HAVE

herb syrup with sage: Use herb syrup with thyme or rosemary (page 206).

why this combination works: Apples and sage are an autumnal match made in heaven, whether baked, roasted, or sipped. The sweetly aromatic juice of apples is tempered by the herbaceous, slightly bitter greenness of sage, so we wanted to turn this winning combo into a drink. We found the best expression of apple as a liquid to come in the form of apple cider. However, apple cider is so concentrated that we needed only ¼ cup (to ¾ cup seltzer) for its apple-iness to shine through the bubbles. We turned to our sweetened herb syrup to infuse the drink with fresh sage flavor (to keep the autumnal theme) without the need for muddling. To balance the sweetness of this drink, we decided to forgo our normal citrus route and instead turned to the on-brand ingredient of apple cider vinegar. Not only did this naturally fermented condiment offer acidity, it also added complexity through secondary notes of apples.

Fill chilled glass halfway with ice. Add apple cider, sage syrup, and vinegar and stir to combine. Add seltzer and, using spoon, gently lift cider mixture from bottom of glass to top to combine. Top with additional ice and garnish with apple slices and sage leaves, if using. Serve.

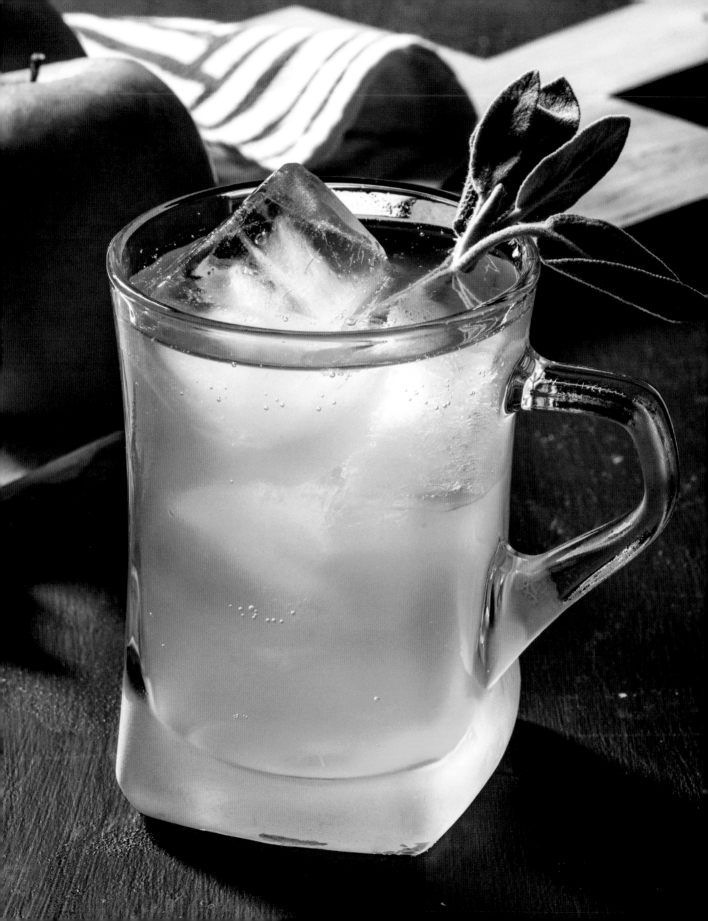

sicilian sunrise

SERVES 1

½ **cup blood orange juice (3 oranges)**

1½ **teaspoons lemon juice**

1 **tablespoon Herb Syrup with tarragon (page 206)**

½ **cup seltzer, chilled**

Tarragon sprig, for garnish (optional)

IF YOU DON'T HAVE

blood oranges: Use navel oranges.

herb syrup with tarragon: Use simple syrup (page 5) or herb syrup with basil (page 206).

why this combination works: Blood oranges are a particularly beautiful and flavorful winter standout, with their peak season being December through April. They are a bit smaller than regular oranges, and they feature prominently in southern Italian (specifically Sicilian) cuisine. When juiced, these oranges make for a striking dark magenta drink with flavor notes of raspberry and just a touch of grapefruit-style bitterness. For our refreshing and flavorful alcohol-free blood orange cocktail, we turned to fresh tarragon, whose anise-licorice notes combine with citrus to form a classic combination that is found in many a Mediterranean dish. Just a tablespoon of the syrup gave us plenty of tarragon flavor, and a touch of lemon juice balanced the sweetness and acidity of the freshly squeezed blood orange juice. Poured over ice and topped with chilled seltzer, our beverage was rich in citrus flavor, with a unique herbal back note and a beautiful color to brighten even the darkest winter day.

Fill chilled glass halfway with ice. Add orange juice, lemon juice, and tarragon syrup and stir to combine. Add seltzer and, using spoon, gently lift juice mixture from bottom of glass to top to combine. Top with additional ice and garnish with tarragon sprig, if using. Serve.

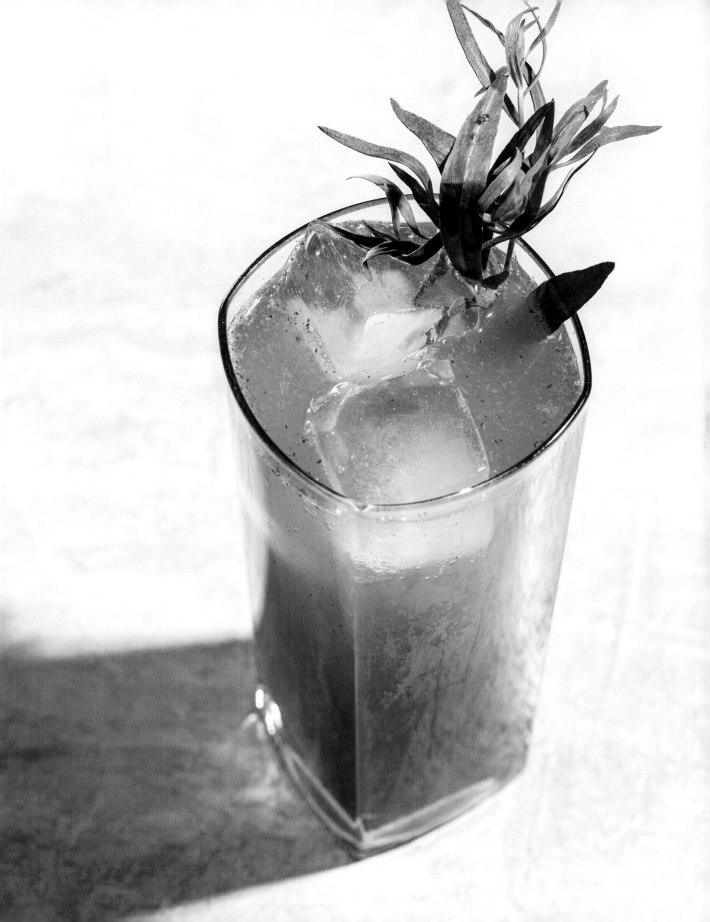

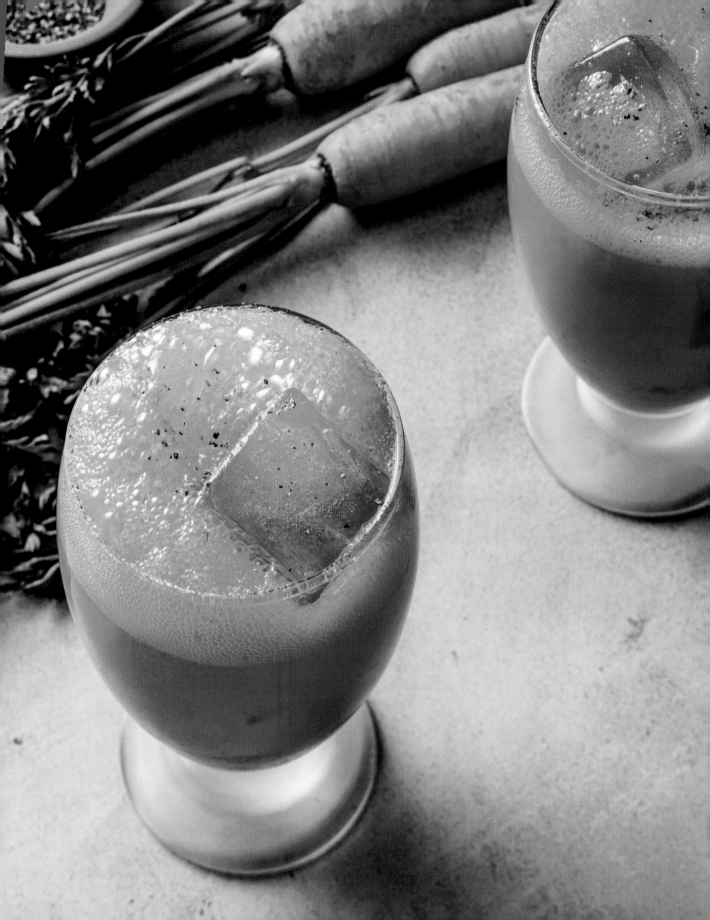

why this combination works: Inspired by cocktails and their delicate balance of flavors, as well as our healthful juices, we wanted to highlight carrot juice in an alcohol-free cocktail. Carrot juice is naturally sweet and earthy and has a striking orange hue. Turmeric is a rhizome known for its punchy and spicy flavor profile. Our Tonic Syrup, made with fresh citrus peel, lemongrass, and cinchona bark, has sweetness and bitterness but also floral notes. Together, these ingredients create an energizing way to enjoy their health benefits. Be sure to use fresh ingredients if possible. Ground turmeric can be substituted, but steer clear of store-bought carrot juice; the flavors are not as complex and detract from the result. We prefer to use our homemade Tonic Syrup (page 204) and seltzer here; however, you can substitute 1¼ cups store-bought tonic water for the syrup and seltzer, if you like.

1. In order listed, process turmeric and carrots through juicer on high speed into 1-cup measuring cup.

2. Fill 2 chilled glasses halfway with ice. Add ½ cup juice, ½ cup seltzer, and 2 tablespoons tonic syrup to each glass. Using spoon, gently lift juice mixture from bottom of glass to top to combine. Top with additional ice and sprinkle with pepper. Serve.

doctor's orders

SERVES 2

1   **(3-inch) piece turmeric root**

1¼ **pound carrots, unpeeled**

1   **cup seltzer, chilled, divided**

¼   **cup Tonic Syrup (page 204), divided**

Black pepper, for garnish

IF YOU DON'T HAVE

turmeric root: Whisk ½ teaspoon ground turmeric into carrot juice.

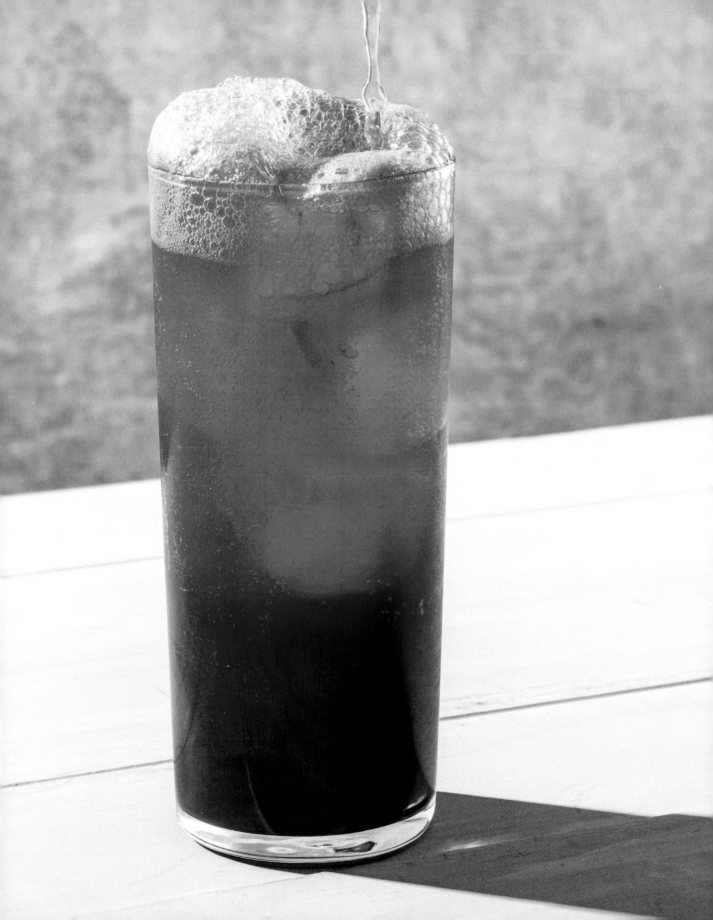

why this combination works: Because we loved the unique vegetable flavors that we uncovered when creating our juice recipes, we wanted to translate some of those ingredients into exciting seltzers. Juices can be combined with seltzers to make lighter, bubblier versions of these good-for-you beverages. To start, we juiced earthy beets for their depth of flavor and rich color, along with the spicy heat of ginger and the sweet acidity of orange. A 2-inch piece of ginger on its own is very strong and overpowering, but it was delectable once diluted by the seltzer. We used a lower ratio of juice to seltzer because the taste of the beets was so potent that it didn't require much to flavor the water and make an enjoyable drink. The inspiration for our drink's name came after we found that the bubbles from the seltzer amplified the foam from the beet juice, creating a massive head of pink foam on top of the drink. For the most dramatic presentation, we recommend using a tall, narrow 12-ounce collins (or highball) glass.

1. On high speed, process ginger, orange, and beets (in that order) though juicer into 1-cup measuring cup.

2. Fill 2 collins glasses with ice. Add ¼ cup juice and ½ cup seltzer to each and let sit for 30 seconds. Slowly pour in ¼ cup seltzer (thick foam will rise above rim). Serve.

beet fizz

SERVES 2

1 **(2-inch) piece ginger, unpeeled**

½ **orange, peeled**

6 **ounces beets, trimmed and halved if larger than 3 inches**

1½ **cups seltzer, chilled, divided**

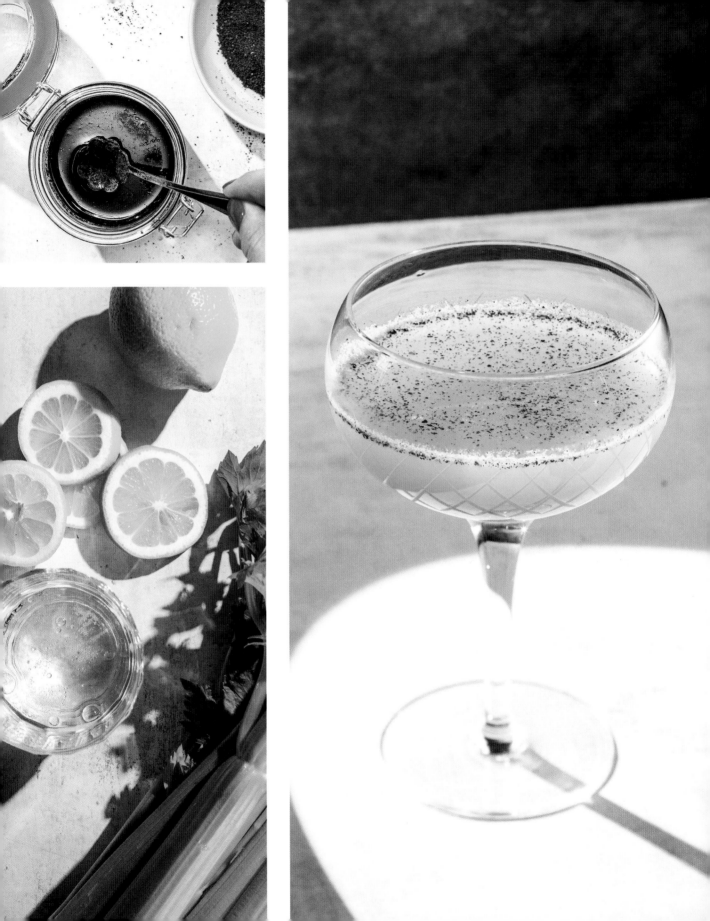

why this combination works: When we found out how deliciously salty-sweet celery turns after juicing, we knew we had the bones of a top-notch alcoholic-free cocktail. Most cocktails are all about the balance of sweet and sour versus bitter and aromatic. We had the naturally bittersweet celery in good order, so we offset that with a slice of lemon for a little spritz of acidity as well as the rich citrus oils contained in the zest. Sumac adds a peppery, berrylike kick to many salads, which makes it a great counter to a vegetable drink. Simply sprinkling it in didn't provide sufficient strength without turning the drink unpalatably gritty, but infusing sumac into a syrup gave us the richly flavored, garnet-hued zing we were after. It layered cleanly into the taste of celery, and a small sprinkle on top lifted the whole drink. This recipe will yield about ½ cup sumac syrup (enough for 6 drinks). Extra syrup can be refrigerated for up to 1 month.

1. for the sumac syrup: Heat sugar, water, and sumac in small saucepan over medium heat, whisking often, until sugar has dissolved, about 5 minutes; do not boil. Let cool completely, about 30 minutes.

2. for the cocktail: On high speed, process lemon and celery (in that order) through juicer into 1-cup measuring cup.

3. Fill 2 glasses with ice. Add ½ cup juice, ½ cup seltzer, and 1 tablespoon sumac syrup to each. Using spoon, gently lift juice mixture from bottom of glass to top to combine. Top with additional ice and sprinkle with sumac. Serve.

celery-sumac sensation

SERVES 2

SUMAC SYRUP

- 6 **tablespoons sugar**
- ¼ **cup water**
- 1½ **tablespoons ground sumac, plus extra for garnish**

COCKTAIL

- 2 **(¼-inch-thick) slices lemon**
- 12 **ounces celery**
- 1 **cup seltzer, chilled, divided**

tonic syrup

Tonic water's characteristic bitterness comes from quinine, an alkaloid extracted from the bark of the tropical cinchona tree. In addition to the many commercial carbonated options, there are also an increasing number of artisanal syrups available for mixing with seltzer to make your own tonic water. We set out to create our own homemade tonic syrup, using fresh ingredients, that would rival any store-bought version. We gently simmered cinchona bark, lemon and lime zest and juice, and lemongrass in water, then added sugar and citric acid (which provided tartness and increased the syrup's shelf life). We let the mixture sit overnight to extract as much flavor as possible before straining out the solids. Unlike commercially produced versions, tonic water made from our syrup has an amber color from the cinchona bark.

tonic syrup

**MAKES 2 CUPS
(ENOUGH FOR 8 SODAS)**

- 2 **cups water**

- 2 **tablespoons (½ ounce) cinchona bark chips**

- 5 **(3-inch) strips lemon zest plus 1 tablespoon juice**

- 4 **(2-inch) strips lime zest plus 1½ teaspoons juice**

- 1 **lemongrass stalk, trimmed to bottom 6 inches and chopped coarse**

    Pinch table salt

- 1 **cup sugar**

- 2 **tablespoons citric acid**

You can purchase cinchona bark chips online or in specialty spice shops; look for ¼-inch chips. You can purchase food-grade citric acid online or in grocery stores that sell canning supplies.

1. Bring water, cinchona bark chips, lemon zest and juice, lime zest and juice, lemongrass, and salt to simmer in medium saucepan over medium-high heat. Reduce heat to low, cover, and cook, stirring occasionally, for 30 minutes.

2. Off heat, stir in sugar and citric acid until dissolved. Cover and let sit for at least 12 hours or up to 24 hours.

3. Set fine-mesh strainer over medium bowl and line with triple layer of cheesecloth. Strain syrup through prepared strainer, pressing on solids to extract as much syrup as possible; discard solids. (Syrup can be refrigerated in airtight container for up to 2 months. Shake gently before using.)

to make tonic water: Add ¾ cup seltzer and ¼ cup tonic syrup to ice-filled glass and stir gently to combine. Top with additional ice and serve.

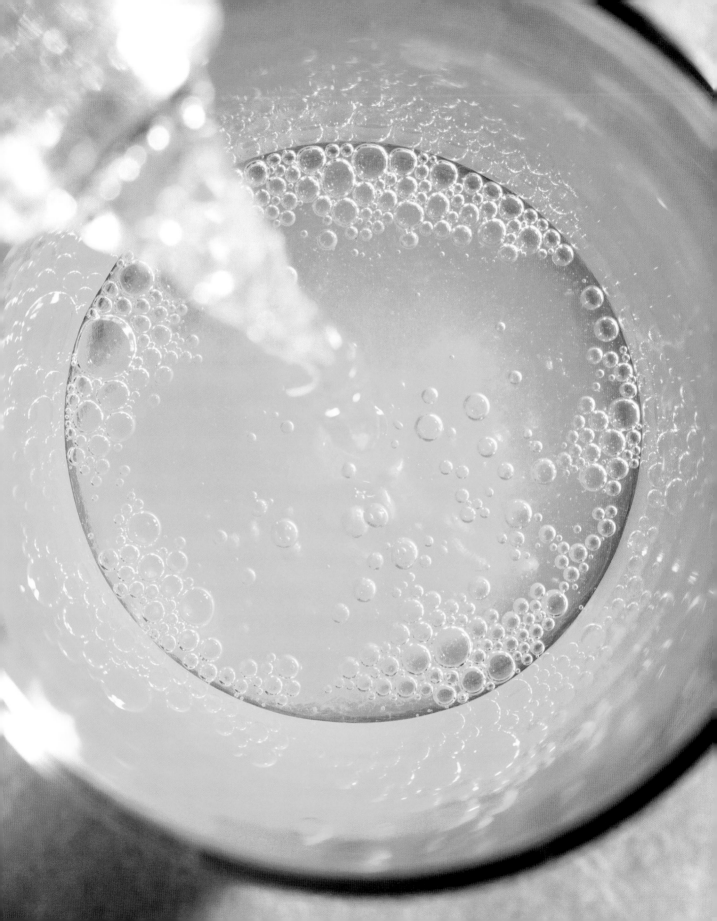

soda syrups

Whether you call it soda or pop, you can still enjoy a favorite drink while being healthy. With these syrups, you can feel good about drinking healthier, homemade soda because you know exactly what went into it—no mystery ingredients. While these syrups still use sugar for sweetness, the amount per serving is quite small when compared to a bottled beverage. These simple syrups make up to 16 servings (depending upon the strength of flavor you prefer) and can easily be stored for up to 1 month.

citrus syrup

**MAKES 1 CUP
(ENOUGH FOR 16 SODAS)**

¾ **cup sugar**

⅔ **cup water**

2 **teaspoons grated grapefruit, lemon, lime, or orange zest**

Heat sugar, water, and zest in small saucepan over medium heat, whisking often, until sugar has dissolved, about 5 minutes; do not boil. Let cool completely, about 30 minutes. Strain syrup through fine-mesh strainer into airtight container; discard solids. (Syrup can be refrigerated for up to 1 month.)

to make flavored soda: Add 1 cup seltzer and 1 to 2 tablespoons flavored syrup to ice-filled glass and stir gently to combine.

VARIATIONS
berry syrup
Substitute 1 cup mashed blueberries, raspberries, or strawberries for citrus zest.

ginger syrup
Substitute 2 tablespoons grated fresh ginger for citrus zest.

herb syrup
Substitute ½ cup fresh herb leaves (basil, dill, mint, sage, or tarragon), 12 fresh thyme sprigs, or 1 fresh rosemary sprig for citrus zest, adding herb after simple syrup is removed from heat.

spiced syrup
Substitute 1 cinnamon stick, 8 lightly crushed allspice berries, and 4 whole cloves for citrus zest.

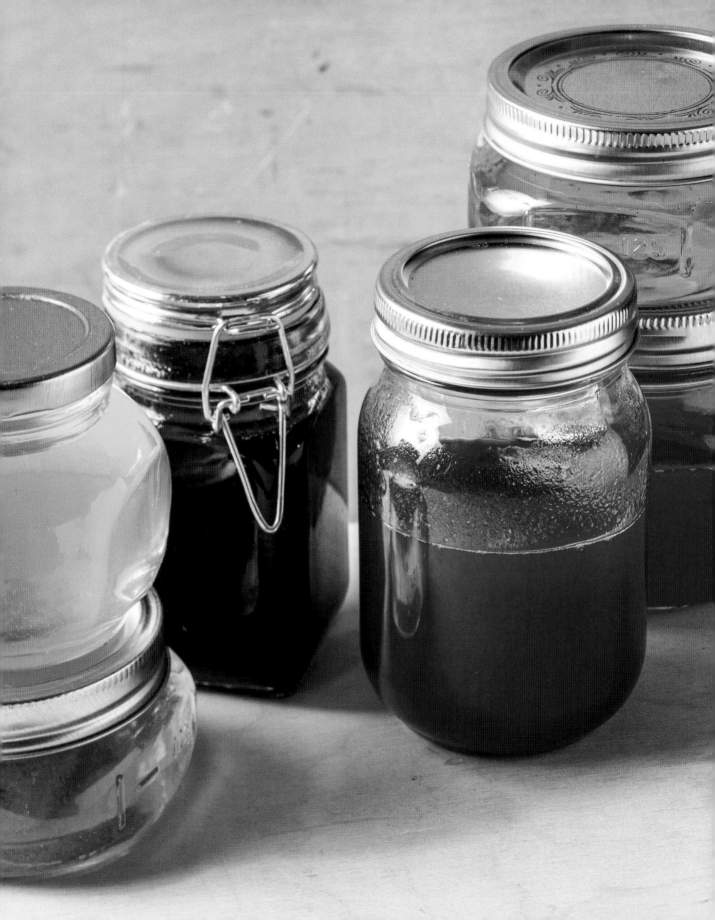

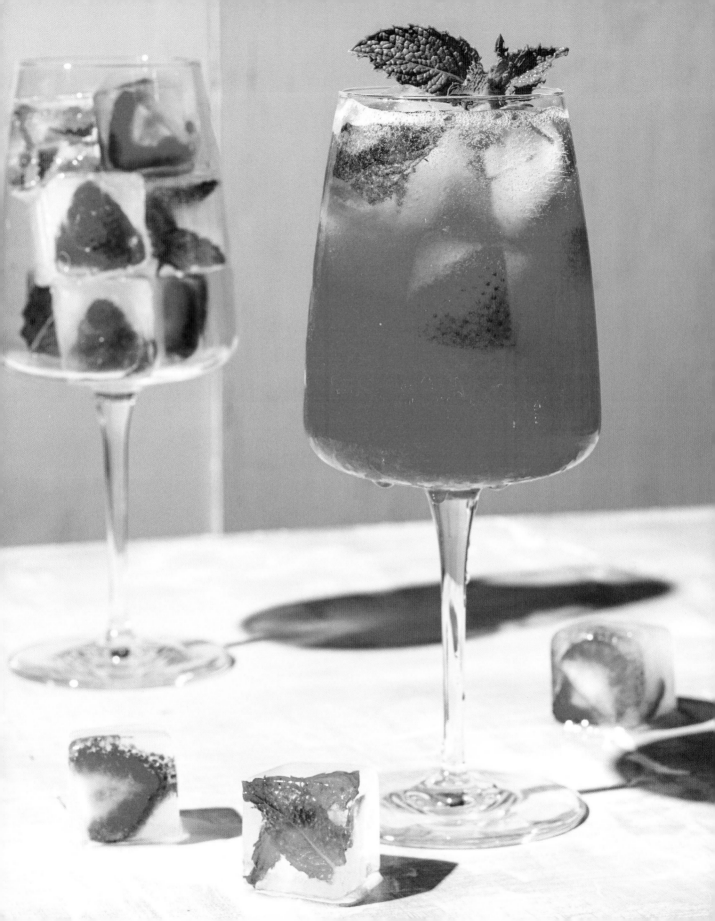

why this combination works: By mixing and matching our soda syrups (page 206), you can create custom blends to satisfy your sweet tooth or wow your friends. There are so many different flavors you can make at home, and this refreshing and sweet combo is one of our favorites. The already sweetened herb and berry syrups combine with seltzer to create a colorful drink that tastes like sparkling, cool strawberry. Other pairings we love are zippy ginger syrup with the slightly sour lime syrup, and our warm spiced syrup with orange syrup. Once you've combined the syrup and seltzer water, it is important to stir the drink gently, so as to not knock out all the bubbles.

Add seltzer, mint syrup, and strawberry syrup to ice-filled glass and stir gently to combine.

VARIATIONS

ginger-lime soda
Substitute 1½ teaspoons Ginger Syrup (page 206) and 1½ teaspoons Citrus Syrup with lime (page 206) for mint syrup and strawberry syrup.

orange-spiced soda
Substitute 2 teaspoons Citrus Syrup with orange (page 206) and 1 teaspoon Spiced Syrup (page 206) for mint syrup and strawberry syrup.

strawberry-mint soda

SERVES 1

1 cup seltzer

2 teaspoons Herb Syrup with mint (page 206)

2 teaspoons Berry Syrup with strawberries (page 206)

shrub syrups

Sweetened vinegar-and-fruit syrups, known as shrubs, date back centuries. The modern version we know is believed to have evolved from the vinegary preserves that American colonists used to keep seasonal fruit. We wanted to develop simple shrub recipes that were bursting with clean, bright, tangy fruit flavor. Berries or peaches (the choice is yours) served as our base, then we simply simmered them with sugar and water until they began to break down. We strained out the solids before adding a dash of white wine vinegar to the syrup. These syrups can make up to 10 sodas and will keep in the fridge for up to 1 month.

mixed berry shrub syrup

MAKES 1¼ CUPS (ENOUGH FOR 10 SODAS)

- 1 **cup blueberries, blackberries, or raspberries, chopped**
- 1 **cup strawberries, hulled and chopped**
- 1 **cup sugar**
- ¼ **cup white wine vinegar**

1. Bring berries and sugar to boil in large saucepan over high heat. Reduce heat to medium-low, cover, and simmer, stirring occasionally, until berries are beginning to break down, 5 to 10 minutes.

2. Remove saucepan from heat and use potato masher to crush berries until uniform in texture. Strain mixture through fine-mesh strainer into medium bowl, pressing on solids to extract as much liquid as possible; discard solids. Whisk in vinegar. (Syrup can be refrigerated for up to 1 month; shake well before using.)

to make shrub soda: Add ¾ cup seltzer and 2 to 4 tablespoons flavored syrup to ice-filled glass and stir gently to combine.

VARIATIONS
cranberry shrub syrup
Substitute 2 cups fresh or frozen cranberries for berries. Add ¾ cup water to saucepan with cranberries.

peach shrub syrup
Substitute 1¾ cups chopped fresh or frozen peaches for berries. Substitute apple cider vinegar for white wine vinegar. Add ¾ cup water to saucepan with peaches.

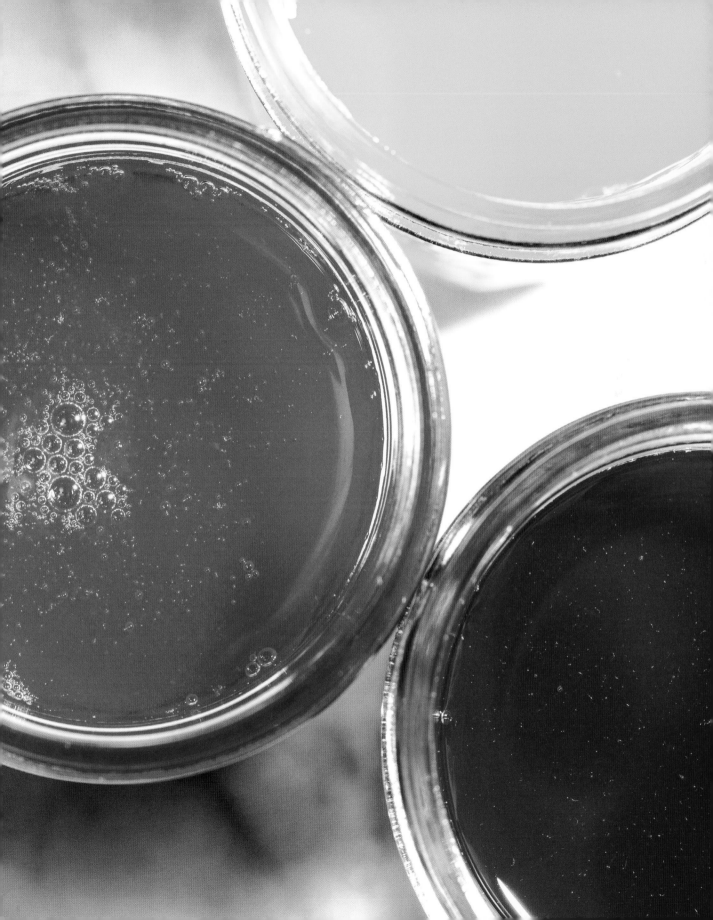

mixed berry shrub soda with mint

SERVES 1

¼ **cup Mixed Berry Shrub Syrup (page 210)**

1 **teaspoon lime juice**

1 **tablespoon fresh mint leaves, plus extra for garnish**

¾ **cup seltzer, chilled**

why this combination works: This homemade soda takes advantage of lime juice, fresh mint leaves, and our versatile mixed berry shrub syrup, which can be made from whatever berries you like the most, for a fresh-tasting, sweet-and-sour soda. Here, the intensely juicy fruit flavor from our berry syrup was brightened and accentuated by the acidity from a splash of fresh lime juice. We mixed these in the bottom of our glass, then added some fresh mint leaves to impart trace notes of their invigorating flavor. Finally, pouring seltzer into our flavored ingredients and gently stirring them together gave us a sparkling and fruity-tasting beverage with subtle hints of mint. The faint color from the berries and the tangy taste will feel like a summery treat and is sure to impress any guest. Garnish with fresh berries if desired.

Add syrup, lime juice, and mint to ice-filled glass and stir to combine. Add seltzer and, using spoon, gently lift shrub mixture from bottom of glass to top to combine. Top with additional ice and garnish with mint leaves. Serve.

VARIATIONS
cranberry shrub soda with lime
Substitute ¼ cup cranberry shrub syrup for mixed berry shrub syrup. Add 1 extra teaspoon lime juice. Omit mint. Garnish with fresh lime twist.

peach shrub soda with lemon
Substitute ¼ cup peach shrub syrup for mixed berry shrub syrup. Substitute 2 teaspoons lemon juice for lime juice. Omit mint. Garnish with fresh peach slice (optional).

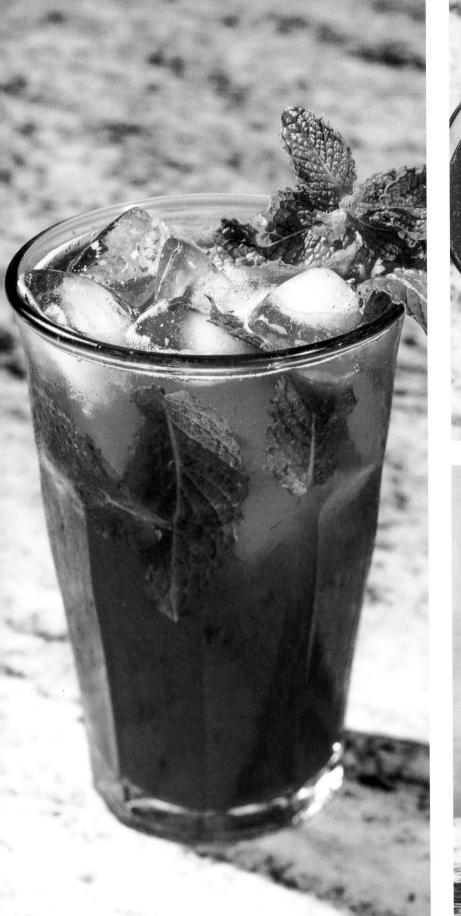
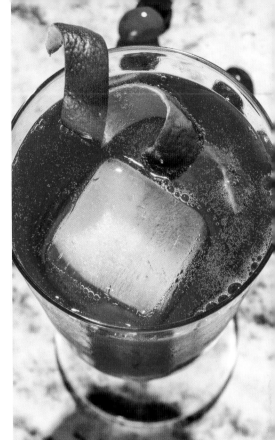
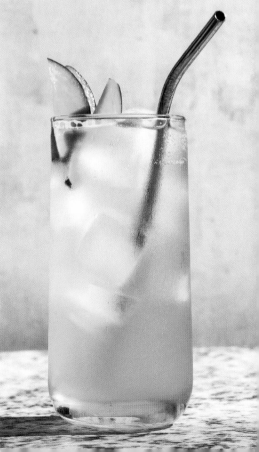

fermented, soaked & simmered

fermenting 101

Fermented drinks are known to have probiotic benefits that can help improve digestive health. Fermenting drinks at home may sound intimidating, but we've worked hard to make it simpler and less prone to failure. (Fermenting is inherently wild, so you can never truly control it.) We spent months developing recipes for trickier beverages such as tepache, kefir, and kombucha that are easy to follow and offer big rewards. While the process of fermentation is inconsistent, we standardized our recipes to make the results as predictable as possible, though outcomes still do vary depending on a number of factors (see below). Besides fermenting, we go deep into soaked and simmered drinks from raw hot chocolate and turmeric milk to nondairy milks and sipping broths.

WHAT TO USE

Throughout this chapter, we use different pieces of equipment, depending on the drink. Glass vessels, such as a 1-gallon wide-mouth Mason jar and a 2-cup Mason jar, are easy to clean and sanitize. Flip-top pint-size bottles for kombucha, called Grolsch-style bottles, are a must. Beyond containers, we use strainers and other stainless-steel, nonreactive materials, which are necessary because they prevent contamination. Additionally, in the test kitchen we use a dye-free, fragrance-free detergent for washing and an iodophor sanitizer, a disinfectant containing iodine (prepared to the manufacturer's instructions), when necessary. If your dishwasher has a sterilization setting, that can be used instead.

SANITATION MATTERS

Cleanliness is super important for any drink you make at home, but especially fermented ones. The ideal environment for fermentation is also ideal for growth of unwanted bacteria and other beverage-spoilers, so sanitation is of utmost importance. You must wash, sanitize, and air-dry all utensils, jars, and bottles that will come in contact with your homemade beverage.

Many factors can affect fermentation. It is largely impacted by temperature and the amount of cultures present, so fermentation rates may vary.

WHERE TO FERMENT

Choose a warm place for your fermenting space. You need a consistent temperature range for your beverage (ideally between 70 and 80 degrees), and the less fluctuation the better. The cooler the environment, the longer the fermentation may take, sometimes never succeeding at all. If the temperature is too high and the process occurs too quickly, there will be less nuanced flavor and you're more likely to overferment and miss the optimal stopping point. Plus, this can lead to a greater production of alcohol.

WHY YOUR WATER MATTERS

During our fermentation experimentation, we tested with tap water, distilled water, spring water, and filtered water. They all worked, but we ended up choosing filtered water or spring water to ensure the best quality outcome. Distilled water lacks minerals, which yeast needs to grow effectively. Additionally, some tap water is highly chlorinated, which is harmful to the microbes, and other tap water may have pathogens, which you don't want to incubate for two weeks in the middle of the temperature danger zone (80 degrees is optimal for growing most good and bad microbes). So filtered or spring water was deemed best for safety and optimal brewing conditions.

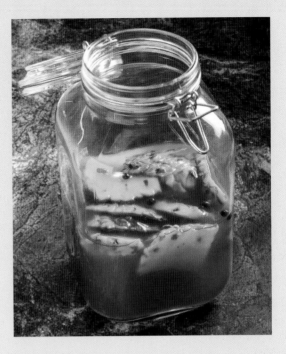

EAT YOUR MISTAKES

The easiest and best way to tell if you have overfermented is by taste. If it is too tart, acidic, and vinegar-forward to enjoy as a drink, you have overfermented. If you happen to overferment your drinks, you can still use what is produced.

kombucha: Kombucha will essentially turn into vinegar, so use it however you would a standard vinegar. Or simmer leftover kombucha in a saucepan until reduced to a sweet syrup to use in alcohol-free cocktails and cocktails.

kefir: This tangy-tasting yogurt-like drink can be used as a sub for buttermilk in dressings or added to any smoothie you want. You can strain it through cheesecloth and make yogurt or labneh (spreadable yogurt cheese).

tepache: It's hardly a mistake if your tepache overferments, because tepache is often mixed with beer, or fermented longer so it becomes more alcoholic. So, while the alcohol level may be more than you bargained for, enjoy it as is or mixed with other alcoholic beverages.

TEPACHE: BRING ON THE FUNK

When tepache starts fermenting, it tastes like a fresh pineapple-forward juice, and as it continues through the process it develops rich caramel undertones. It also gains a slightly musky note that is reminiscent of sour hard cider. You can still taste the pineapple, but it is less sweet and a little more funky. That is when you know it is ready.

DRINK RESPONSIBLY

The creation of alcohol occurs naturally as a by-product during the fermentation process. The fermented beverages in this chapter can contain between 0.5 and 3 percent alcohol by volume depending on duration of fermentation time and ingredients used. Kefir is at the lower end of the range, and tepache and kombucha are at the higher end. If a drink overferments, it can lead to a greater percentage of alcohol by volume. In Mexico, there are versions of tepache that are intentionally made more alcoholic by fermenting them longer.

making kombucha at home

We experimented and tested and retested all of the variables and a variety of methods and equipment to develop the easiest-to-follow, hardest-to-mess-up recipe for homemade kombucha. Making your own kombucha may seem daunting, but it's as simple as combining water, tea, a bit of sugar, and already mature kombucha to create an endless and economical supply at home. Everyone in the test kitchen who tested the recipe, all first-time drink fermenters, were surprised by how easy it was—and by how much better the home-brewed kombucha tasted than store-bought. While the fear of botulism is a common concern when fermenting, kombucha is too acidic for botulism to grow; additonally, botulism spores need an anaerobic (low- or no-oxygen) environment, and plenty of oxygen gets through the coffee filter over the top of the jar.

making your first batch

For your first batch, we recommend purchasing a kombucha starter, which contains the mature kombucha and kombucha pellicle (the jelly-like culture of bacteria and yeasts that acts as a starter), through an online retailer. Amounts of mature kombucha and pellicle vary by manufacturer. We call for the least amount necessary for success; however, you should include the entire amount of starter if a greater amount is provided for your initial batch. If your kombucha starter came with less than ½ cup of mature kombucha, make up the difference with unpasteurized, unflavored store-bought kombucha.

"HOW DO I KNOW WHEN MY KOMBUCHA IS READY?"

Knowing when the correct sweet-acidic balance has been achieved during the fermentation process can be challenging for the novice brewer. To help calibrate your palate, we created a vinegar-sugar mixture to use as a benchmark. Each time you plan to check the maturity of your kombucha, first take a small sip of the calibrator to remind yourself of the target sweetness and acidity.

HOW TO MAKE YOUR KOMBUCHA CALIBRATOR

This calibrator is easier to use and a better estimator of what you are tasting than a pH meter or strips. Whisk 1 cup water, 1½ teaspoons sugar, and 4 teaspoons apple cider vinegar together in bowl; transfer to storage container. (Mixture can be refrigerated for up to 2 weeks.)

best practices

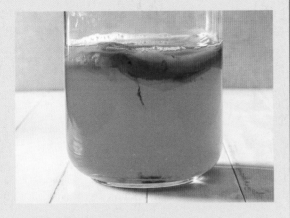

- Starting a fresh batch of kombucha with a portion of mature kombucha not only inoculates the brew with the pellicle, but it also lowers its pH, making it inhospitable to unwanted microbes. Aside from good hygiene, your best defense against mold is adequate acidification. If you want reassurance that you have acidified your sweetened tea sufficiently, use pH strips to verify that the pH of your starting brew is below 4. If it is not, add more mature kombucha or distilled white vinegar (in ½-teaspoon increments) until the pH registers below 4.

- As mentioned, fermentation is an inconsistent process, so results do vary. When making sparkling kombucha, you may find that the time frames listed do not exactly match your experience. In these cases, adjust the fermentation time by a day or two on your next batch.

- When opening sparkling kombucha, it's best to make sure your bottles are well chilled. This will reduce the chance of bottles foaming over. Just in case, open the bottles slowly, with caps pointed away from you, in a safe environment.

SHARING YOUR PELLICLE

The pellicle, often called a SCOBY (symbiotic culture of bacteria and yeast), refers to the jellyfish-like membrane or skin that forms on the surface of the fermenting kombucha. This can be split and shared with others to make more kombucha, as the pellicle forms a new layer every time it's disturbed. Using gloved (or very clean) hands, you can pull apart the individual layers. We recommend storing the pellicle in 1 cup of kombucha at room temperature to guarantee you have at least ¾ cup of mature kombucha to start your next batch. You can store the pellicle and mature kombucha for up to 2 weeks at room temperature.

BOTTLING KOMBUCHA

Our favorite containers for putting up kombucha are round bottles called Grolsch-style. They have flip-top lids and rubber gaskets that are pressure rated. These bottles are especially important when doing a second fermentation for kombucha because the carbonation builds to create a sparkling drink, and they have a safety gasket to help keep the glass bottle from exploding. If too much gas builds up, it will pop and release to let out some gas from the bottle. Do not use square bottles, as they are weaker and susceptible to shattering under pressure. Plastic soda bottles and recycled store-bought kombucha bottles work well too.

the ins and outs of kefir

Kefir grains are a culture of bacteria and yeast that ferment milk into a thickened beverage known as milk kefir. Fresh kefir grains resemble cottage cheese and are often coated in a layer called kefiran that, among other things, gives milk kefir its gel-like consistency. Package sizes and instructions for kefir grains can vary by manufacturer, so we tested multiple kinds of kefir grains and followed their activation instructions step by step to find the best common method that would work for all of them. Our yield is smaller than most because the kefir fermentation cycle is short and produces a new batch every day, so we aimed to avoid waste (though the recipe can be doubled if you prefer). Dehydrated kefir grains will not work in this recipe. Milk that is ultra-high temperature (UHT) pasteurized is unsuitable for culturing and will not work for this recipe. Metallic containers are not recommended for storage as they affect the kefir grains, and the acidic kefir can ruin them. When straining and stirring, be sure to use rubber utensils and stainless-steel or nylon mesh strainers.

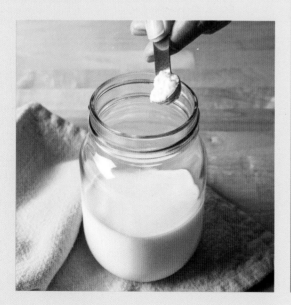

TROUBLESHOOTING KEFIR FERMENTATION

Visual cues are key here. Once properly fermented and ready to strain, the milk kefir will have thickened and gelled (easy to see if you gently tilt the jar).

- **underfermented:** The milk and grains have not thickened or gelled and the mixture has not achieved kefir's pleasantly yeasty and sour smell within the prescribed fermentation time. Increasing the ambient room temperature a few degrees or doubling the amount of grains used in step 2 will speed up the fermentation cycle.

- **overfermented:** There is a noticeable separation of the whey from the milk curd in step 2 of the recipe. Decreasing the ambient room temperature or halving the amount of grains will slow down the fermentation cycle.

SHARING AND STORING ACTIVATED KEFIR GRAINS

When making kefir, you end up with more grains than you need after activation, plus the process of fermentation produces excess kefir grains over time. Unused grains after the activation stage can be shared or stored in the refrigerator or freezer.

- **refrigerate:** Store grains in an airtight jar with enough milk to submerge the grains (about 1 cup of milk for every 1 tablespoon of grains) for up to 2 weeks. To make kefir with refrigerated grains, skip reactivation and continue with step 2 of the recipe.

- **freeze:** Rinse the grains with filtered water, pat dry, toss with dry milk powder (1 tablespoon for every 1 tablespoon of grains), and store in a freezer bag with the air pressed out for up to 6 months. To make kefir with frozen grains, start recipe with one 36-hour reactivation period before proceeding to step 2.

soaking & simmering 101

Soaking and simmering drinks such as Old-Fashioned Mulled Cider (page 235) or Raw Hot Chocolate (page 230) is a great way to gently infuse flavors into a warm drink. These beverages feel almost magical in their creation because ingredients are combined in a saucepan and easily brewed to a delicious result. A great example of this kind of drink is one of our sipping broths, which have grown in popularity as a nutritious beverage. A broth is a great way to start off your morning on a lighter note or get some liquid calories and protein elsewhere in your day.

making nondairy milks

People turn to alternative milks for any number of dietary or health reasons, but store-bought versions typically have stabilizers and added sugars, detracting from their overall healthful nature. We worked to limit the ingredient list to only the necessary items so you know exactly what you're getting when you make our oat, almond, soy, or rice milk. Plus, they are an inexpensive way to make in large quantities. You can substitute them for dairy milk wherever you see fit in smoothies, lattes, overnight oats, baking, and more.

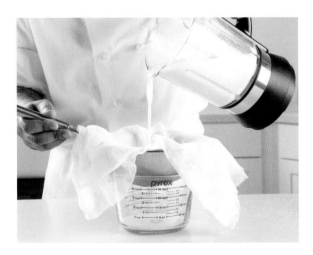

broths

STORING BROTHS

Sipping broths can be stored for up to 4 days in the fridge or up to 1 month in the freezer. Freeze them in single servings for when you just want one glass. Reheat gently to enjoy.

FLAVOR YOUR BROTH

Try one of these flavoring ideas with either the chicken or beef broth when you want to change things up.

chipotle-inspired: Add 1 tablespoon canned chipotle chile and adobo sauce with water in step 2. Add ½ cup fresh cilantro during the last 5 minutes of simmering.

pho-inspired: Add 1 cinnamon stick, 2 whole cloves, one 4-inch piece fresh ginger sliced into rounds, and 4 star anise pods with water in step 2. Once strained, stir in 2 to 4 tablespoons fish sauce.

Provençal-inspired: Add 2 sprigs fresh rosemary, 5 sprigs fresh thyme, 3 crushed garlic cloves, two 3-inch strips orange zest, and 1 rinsed and minced anchovy fillet with water in step 2.

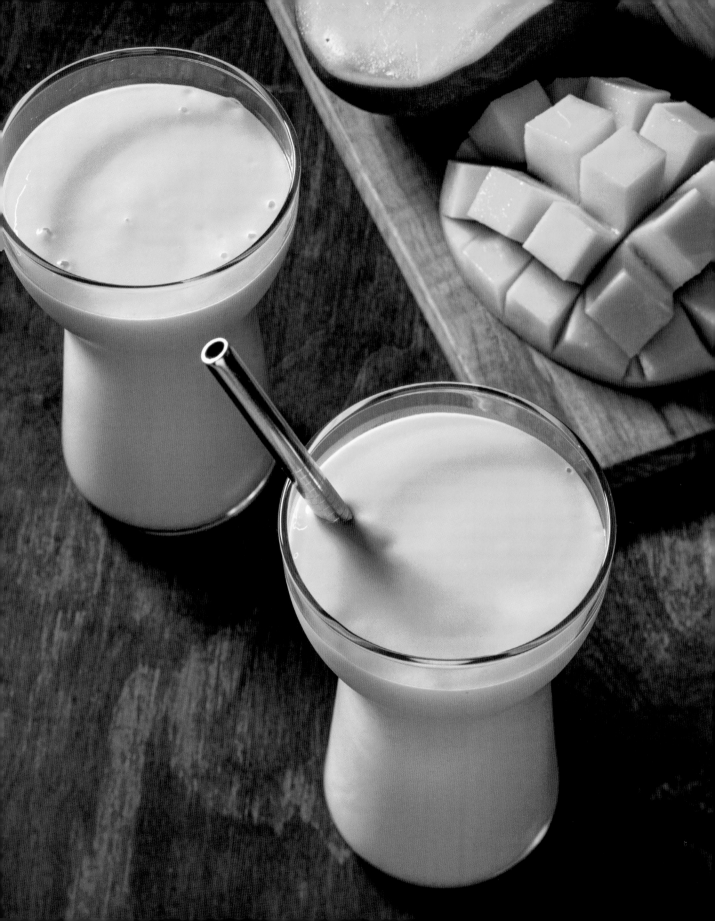

why this combination works: Lassi is a refreshing, creamy, yogurt-forward drink with origins in North Indian cuisine. It is enjoyed for its delicious flavor and also as a support for digestive health due to its yogurt base. To make it, yogurt is blended with water, spices, and other ingredients. Lassis come in many varieties, with mango-flavored one of the most popular around the world. We found that the best mango lassi recipe required a generous amount of fruit; fortunately, frozen mango is convenient, fresh-tasting, and widely available. In addition to the fruit, we liked the full flavor of whole-milk yogurt (though low-fat and nonfat yogurt made reasonably good lassis as well). To keep the drink from becoming unpleasantly thick, we added water to the blender to thin it. For sweetness, we liked the floral notes of honey and found that a pinch of salt and a squeeze of lime juice perked up the tropical mango flavor. We prefer this drink strained for a supersmooth finish, but this step is optional.

In order listed, add all ingredients to blender and process on low speed until mixture is combined but still coarse in texture, about 10 seconds, scraping down sides of blender jar as needed. Gradually increase speed to high and process until completely smooth, about 1 minute. Adjust consistency with extra water as needed. Strain mixture through fine-mesh strainer into pitcher, pressing on solids to extract as much liquid as possible; discard solids. Serve over ice. (Mango lassi can be refrigerated for up to 1 day; stir to recombine before serving.)

mango lassi

SERVES 4 TO 6

4 **cups frozen mango chunks**

2½ **cups plain dairy or plant-based yogurt**

1 **cup water, plus extra as needed**

2 **tablespoons honey**

2 **teaspoons lime juice**

⅛ **teaspoon table salt**

IF YOU DON'T HAVE

frozen mango: Use fresh mango or fresh or frozen pineapple.

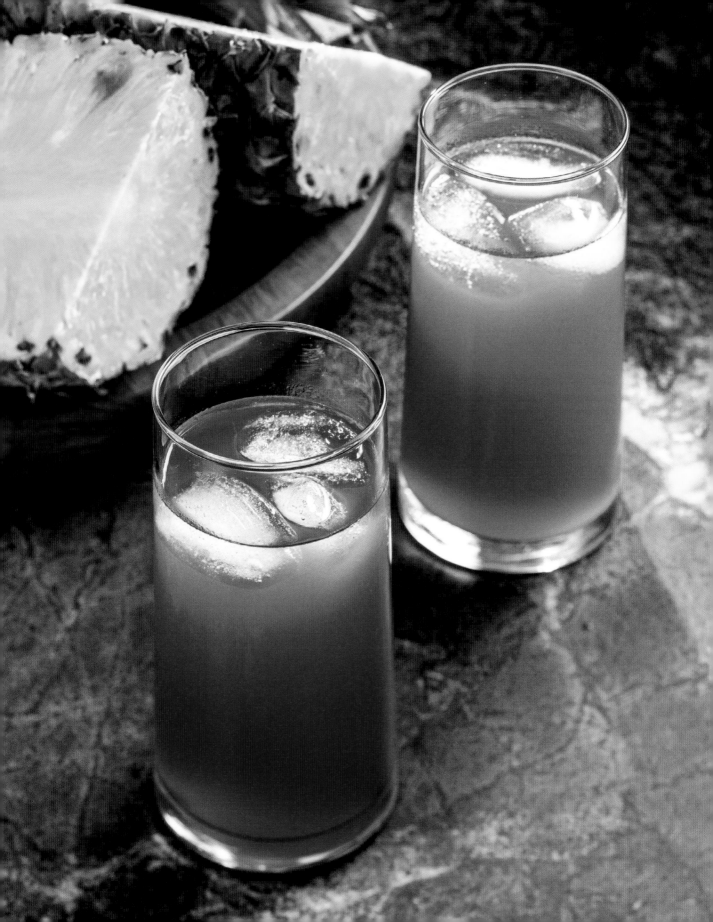

why this combination works: Tepache is a spiced and fruity fermented Mexican beverage that is easy to make at home and does not require the addition of cultures. We decided to make our version as simple as possible by using pineapple peels, cinnamon, and the iconic piloncillo. Piloncillo, also known as panela or panocha, is an unrefined cane sugar used throughout Central and South America. It is traditionally used in tepache and adds rich, caramel-like sweetness. Technique and temperature are of utmost importance to ensure proper and safe fermentation of this recipe. We submerged all ingredients in filtered water with the assistance of parchment paper and a makeshift weight made from a water-filled zipper-lock bag. Maintaining a temperature range from 72 to 75 degrees was also crucial, as any less and the tepache will not ferment. We recommend using a serrated knife to break the piloncillo into smaller pieces for accurate measurement. For more information on sanitizing your equipment, see page 216. You will need a 1-gallon wide-mouth glass jar for this recipe.

1. Discard pineapple crown and peel pineapple. Cut peels into rough 3-inch pieces and set aside; enjoy pineapple flesh separately. Cut out parchment paper round to match diameter of 1-gallon wide-mouth jar.

2. Heat piloncillo, 1 cup spring or filtered tap water, cinnamon stick, and allspice berries (if using) in large saucepan over medium-high heat until piloncillo has dissolved, about 5 minutes. Add pineapple peels, piloncillo syrup, and 4 cups room-temperature spring or filtered tap water to 1-gallon wide-mouth jar and stir to combine. Press parchment round flush against surface of peels. Fill 1-quart zipper-lock bag with 1 cup water, squeeze out air, and seal well. Place bag of water on top of parchment and gently press down to submerge pineapple. Cover jar with large coffee filter or triple layer of cheesecloth and secure with rubber band. Place jar in 72- to 75-degree location away from direct sunlight and let ferment for 3 to 5 days.

3. After 3 days, taste tepache daily until it has reached desired flavor. Beverage should be fruit-forward with caramel and spice undertones and have mild fermented flavor, with slight effervescence.

4. When tepache has reached desired flavor, strain liquid through fine-mesh strainer into storage container; discard solids. Chill tepache for at least 1 hour or up to 1 week. Serve over ice.

tepache

SERVES 4 TO 6

1 pineapple, rinsed

4½ ounces piloncillo, broken up into small pieces (½ cup packed)

1 cinnamon stick

½ teaspoon allspice berries (optional)

IF YOU DON'T HAVE

piloncillo: Use turbinado (such as Sugar in the Raw) or demerara sugar.

milk kefir

SERVES 1

**4–5 cups whole milk, divided,
plus extra as needed**

**1 (¼-ounce) package live
kefir culture**

why this combination works: Milk kefir, made from fermented dairy and kefir grains, is a slightly fizzy, tart, and creamy probiotic drink that is good for your gut health. Milk kefir grains contain bacteria and yeast and, as a result, have higher amounts of probiotics when compared to yogurt. These grains work to culture dairy milk in a matter of only 24 hours, so we made a recipe that produces 1 cup of kefir a day. During shipping, the grains are starved of food (lactose from milk) and the bacteria balances can be thrown off, so it is important to activate them upon arrival. The kefir grains need time to reacquaint to their new environment and build up to their full potential to provide a balanced beverage—slightly yeasty tasting but sour and satisfying like yogurt. We rounded out our testing by trying different milk fat percentages and found that any dairy milk will produce a delicious kefir beverage, but we preferred the thick and rich texture of whole milk. Package sizes for kefir grains can vary by manufacturer. We call for the least amount necessary for success; however, you should include the entire amount of kefir grains in step 1 if a greater amount is provided. For more information on making kefir, see page 220. You will need a 2-cup glass jar with lid for this recipe. Your kefir jar should be covered well but loosely. We find inverting the lid of a Mason jar before sealing with the screw top is an easy way to create a covered but breathable environment for the kefir. This recipe can easily be doubled.

1. to activate kefir: Combine 1 cup milk and kefir grains with their packing liquid in 2-cup glass jar. Cover loosely with lid, place in 68- to 72-degree location away from direct sunlight, and let ferment for 36 hours.

2. Strain mixture through fine-mesh strainer; reserve grains and discard milk. Clean jar. Combine reserved grains and 1 cup fresh milk in now-empty jar, place in 68- to 72-degree location away from direct sunlight, and let ferment for 24 hours. Repeat straining and refreshing grain and milk mixture until milk lightly sours and thickens to buttermilk consistency within 24-hour period, 1 to 2 more times. Strain mixture, reserving activated kefir grains and discarding milk.

3. to make kefir: Combine ⅛ teaspoon activated kefir grains and 1 cup fresh milk in clean jar. Cover loosely with lid, place in 68- to 72-degree location away from direct sunlight, and let ferment until milk lightly sours and thickens to buttermilk consistency, about 24 hours. Store remaining activated kefir grains for later use.

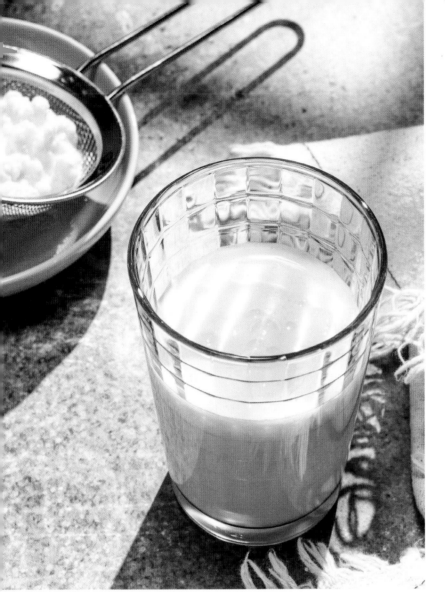

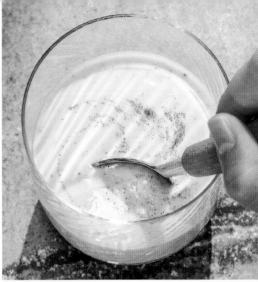

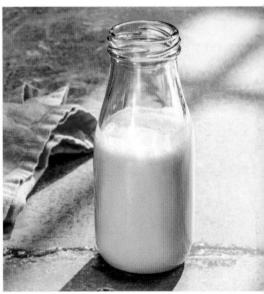

Kefir should not show signs of separation within fermentation cycle; if so, it has overfermented. (See Troubleshooting Kefir Fermentation and Sharing and Storing Activated Kefir Grains on page 220.)

4. Strain kefir through fine-mesh strainer into serving glass or storage container, gently stirring mixture to help separate grains from kefir; reserve grains. Serve or refrigerate kefir for up to 3 days.

5. to make future batches of kefir: Repeat recipe from step 3, using reserved kefir grains. The grains will increase in volume over multiple batches of kefir; we recommend sharing, storing, or discarding excess grains once they measure over ⅛ teaspoon.

VARIATIONS
milk kefir with vanilla
Stir ½ teaspoon vanilla extract into strained kefir until fully combined.

milk kefir with maple and cinnamon
Stir 1 tablespoon maple syrup and ¼ teaspoon ground cinnamon into strained kefir until fully combined.

milk kefir with fruit preserves
Stir 1 tablespoon fruit preserves into strained kefir until fully combined.

kombucha

SERVES 4 TO 6
(MAKES 1½ QUARTS)

8 cups spring or filtered tap water, room temperature, divided

2 tablespoons loose-leaf black or green tea

½ cup (3½ ounces) sugar

¾ cup mature kombucha plus 1 ounce kombucha pellicle

3 tablespoons Simple Syrup (page 5; optional)

IF YOU DON'T HAVE

loose-leaf tea: Use 4 tea bags.

why this combination works: It is startlingly easy and economical to make kombucha at home: Just add sweetened, cooled tea to mature kombucha and allow it to ferment in a warm environment. It's revered for its health benefits, but we love it most for its transformation from syrupy, strong tea to an effervescent, deeply delicious, and refreshing drink. You can consume your kombucha either as a still beverage or let it undergo a secondary fermentation in the bottle to become a sparkling one. This is an ideal time to introduce additional flavorings, although good kombucha tastes fantastic in its pure form. The variation possibilities are endless and ripe for experimentation, whether you want to turn it gingery and blue or try a spicy pineapple version. Once you have mature kombucha and some simple equipment, you'll have all you need to make a consistently satisfying drink. For more information on kombucha making, see pages 218–219. You will need a 1-gallon wide-mouth glass jar and three 16-ounce glass bottles with caps for this recipe.

1. Bring 2 cups water to boil in small saucepan over high heat; remove from heat. (If steeping green tea, allow boiled water to cool to 175 degrees.) Using reusable tea infuser or disposable tea bag, steep tea in water for 5 minutes (if using black tea) or 3 minutes (if using green tea). Discard tea. Whisk in sugar until dissolved.

2. Add sweetened tea and remaining 6 cups water to 1-gallon wide-mouth jar and stir to combine (mixture should be less than 100 degrees; let cool if necessary before proceeding). Stir in mature kombucha and pellicle. Cover jar with large coffee filter and secure with rubber band. Place jar in 73- to 83-degree location away from direct sunlight and let ferment for 6 days. After 6 days, taste kombucha daily until it has reached desired flavor (see "How do I know when my kombucha is ready?" on page 218; this may take up to 8 days longer.)

3. When kombucha has reached desired flavor, transfer pellicle to bowl, using tongs or slotted spoon, along with ¾ cup mature kombucha; set aside. Stir remaining kombucha to recombine.

4a. for still kombucha: Using funnel and ladle, divide kombucha evenly among three 16-ounce bottles, filling each bottle to within 1 inch of top. (Enjoy excess kombucha immediately or refrigerate in separate small container.) Secure bottle caps and refrigerate until chilled, at least 1 hour or up to 1 month. Serve.

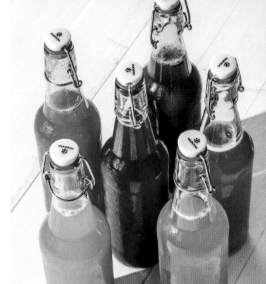

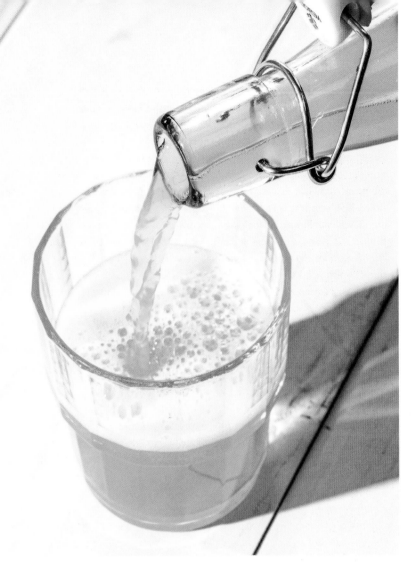

4b. for sparkling kombucha: Using funnel and ladle, fill three 16-ounce bottles halfway with kombucha, add 1 tablespoon simple syrup, and top with remaining kombucha to within 1 inch of top. (Enjoy excess kombucha immediately or refrigerate in separate small container.) Secure bottle caps and gently shake to combine ingredients. Store bottles in 73- to 83-degree location away from direct sunlight for 7 days to carbonate. Refrigerate carbonated kombucha until chilled, at least 1 hour or up to 1 month. Serve, opening bottles slowly to prevent foaming.

5. to make future batches of kombucha: Repeat recipe, using reserved pellicle and mature kombucha in step 2. The pellicle will continue to increase in size over multiple batches of kombucha; we recommend sharing or discarding excess pellicle once it weighs over 5 ounces (see Sharing Your Pellicle on page 219).

VARIATIONS

sparkling blue-ginger lime kombucha

Add 1 teaspoon (¼-inch) dried ginger pieces, 1 teaspoon blue or green spirulina (optional), and ¼ teaspoon grated lime zest to each bottle with simple syrup in step 4b. Reduce carbonating time to 5 days.

sparkling spicy pineapple kombucha

Process 8 ounces thawed frozen organic pineapple chunks and 1 tablespoon minced, seeded Fresno peppers in blender until smooth, about 1 minute. Strain mixture through fine-mesh strainer into small bowl, pressing on solids to extract as much juice as possible; discard solids. Substitute ¼ cup pineapple puree for simple syrup in each bottle in step 4b. Reduce carbonating time to 5 days.

sparkling mixed berry kombucha

Process 8 ounces thawed frozen organic mixed berries in blender until smooth, about 1 minute. Strain mixture through fine-mesh strainer into small bowl, pressing on solids to extract as much juice as possible; discard solids and stir in ½ teaspoon vanilla extract (optional). Substitute ¼ cup berry puree for simple syrup in each bottle in step 4b. Reduce carbonating time to 5 days.

raw hot chocolate

SERVES 4

½ **vanilla bean**

2½ **cups dairy or plant-based milk**

3 **pitted dates**

½ **cup cacao nibs**

why this combination works: Inspired by hot cacao beverages enjoyed by ancient Mayan society, we wanted to make a decadent-tasting hot chocolate that used no added processed sugar at all. We infused our beverage with chocolaty flavor by blooming cacao nibs in milk alongside vanilla beans, whose floral and aromatic notes nicely complemented the complexity of the cacao. To give our drink some unrefined sweetness, we added pitted dates to our simmered mixture, which allowed the dates to soften enough for blending while imparting a honeyed and fruity flavor. After simmering, we blended the still-warm mixture and strained it to remove distracting particulates for smooth sipping. We took care to strain the mixture gently and avoided pressing on the solids, as this resulted in a slightly bitter drink. Our hot chocolate was delectably rich without being overwhelmingly sweet.

1. Cut vanilla bean in half lengthwise. Using tip of paring knife, scrape out seeds. Bring vanilla seeds and bean, milk, dates, and cacao nibs to simmer over medium-high heat in medium saucepan and cook, stirring occasionally, until dates soften and flavors meld, about 5 minutes.

2. Carefully transfer cacao mixture to blender and process until smooth, about 1 minute. Strain mixture through fine-mesh strainer into serving mugs, discarding solids. Serve.

VARIATIONS
raw hot chocolate with ancho chile
Add ½ teaspoon ground ancho chile to saucepan with remaining ingredients in step 1.

raw hot chocolate with orange
Add 1 teaspoon grated orange zest to saucepan with remaining ingredients in step 1.

IF YOU DON'T HAVE

vanilla bean: Use ¼ teaspoon vanilla extract.

cacao nibs: Use ½ cup unsweetened cocoa powder.

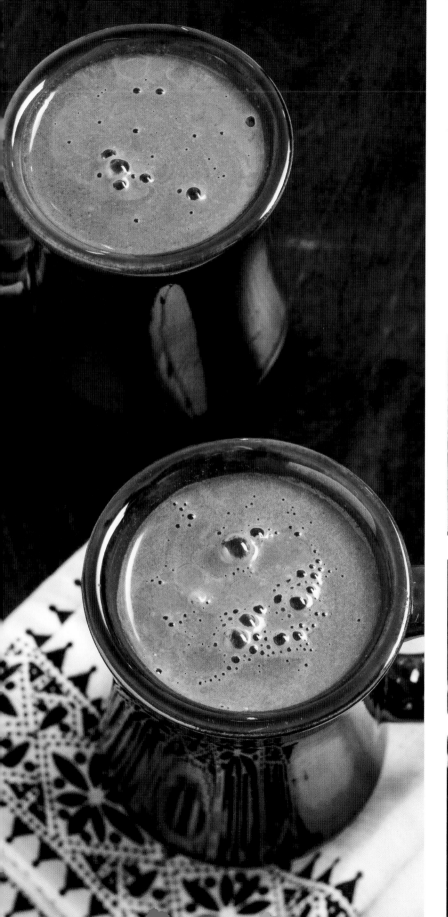
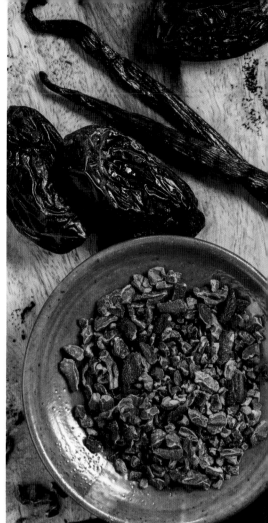
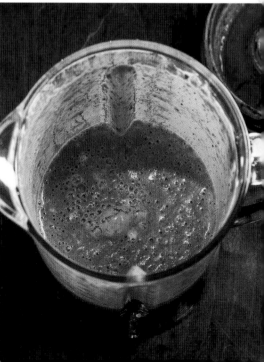

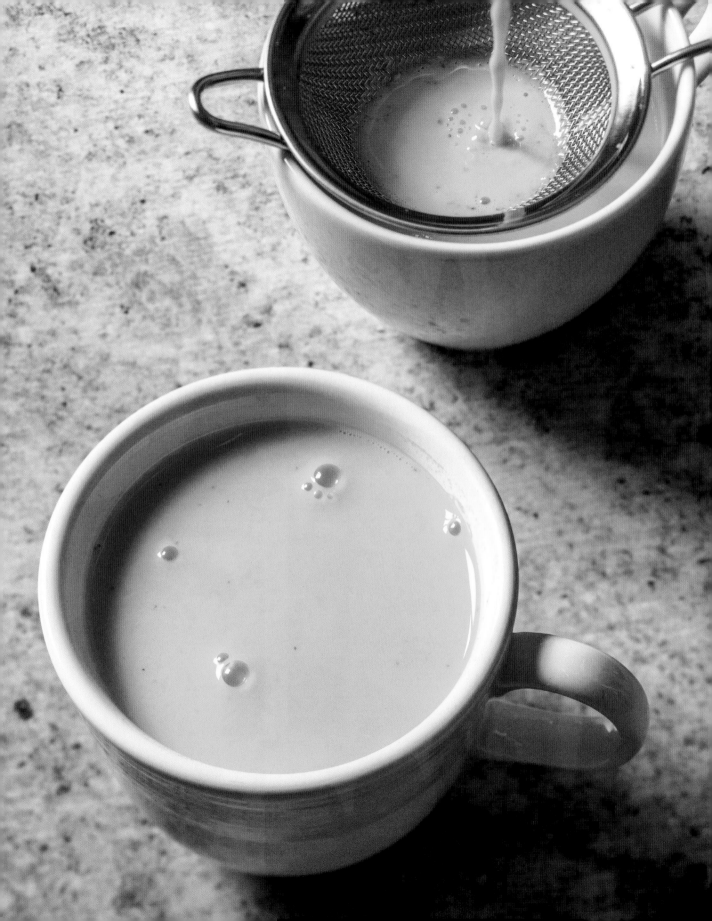

why this combination works: Haldhicha dudh (in the Marathi language of Western India) is a traditional beverage that is used to soothe people when they have a cold or cough. Translated as "turmeric milk," haldhicha dudh combines turmeric with heated sweetened milk. When developing the proper proportions for our recipe, we relied on the advice of our colleague Kaumudi Marathé who grew up with the drink. Because fresh turmeric is seasonal, this drink is instead made with ground turmeric so that it can be enjoyed year-round. Turmeric is a spice that's sensitive to temperature, so we whisked it into the milk off heat to allow it to bloom without overcooking and tasting bitter. We tested a wide range of turmeric amounts and landed on 2 teaspoons—any more and the drink became gritty and tannic (like oversteeped tea), and any less resulted in a too dairy-forward drink. Instead of sugar, we sweetened our milk with honey because it balanced the earthy turmeric while providing a more natural flavor. We enjoyed trying out additional ingredients that paired nicely with the turmeric and found black pepper and ginger to be exciting add-ins thanks to their invigorating flavors. Once we added additional aromatics, a short steep time was necessary to draw out their flavor.

Bring milk to simmer in small saucepan over medium-high heat. Off heat, whisk in turmeric and honey until fully combined. Strain into serving mugs, discarding solids. Serve.

VARIATIONS
haldhicha dudh with black pepper
Add 1 teaspoon cracked black peppercorns with turmeric and honey. Let steep, covered, for 5 minutes before straining and serving.

haldhicha dudh with ginger
Add 1 teaspoon grated fresh ginger with turmeric and honey. Let steep, covered, for 5 minutes before straining and serving.

haldhicha dudh

SERVES 2

2 cups whole milk

2 teaspoons ground turmeric

2 teaspoons honey

IF YOU DON'T HAVE

whole milk: Other varieties of dairy and plant-based milk can be used; we especially like oat milk.

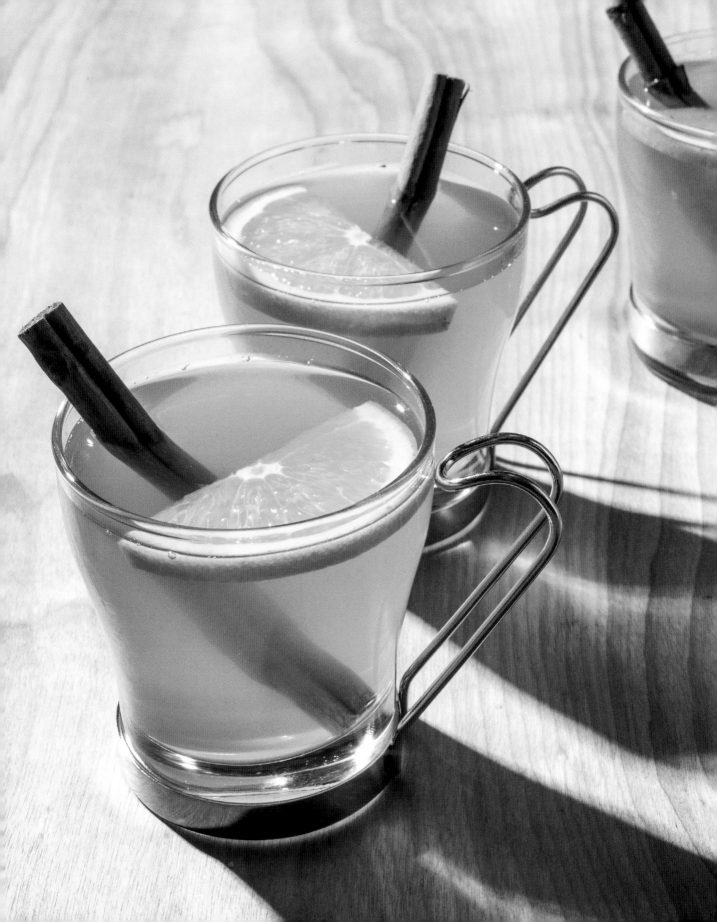

why this combination works: The process of mulling—a term that most often refers to steeping assorted spices, herbs, and citrus fruits in heated red or white wine—can be applied to apple cider to create a warm and autumnal-feeling drink. More often than not, store-bought mulling spices are reminiscent of potpourri, so we wanted to make our own blend that would add spice to cider without overdoing it. One thing became very clear: Less is more. The recipes that called for packing the whole spice cabinet into the pot produced harsh, unpleasant cider. We preferred fewer spices so the flavors of each, and that of the cider, came through clearly. Cinnamon and cloves brought classic holiday flavors, while coriander added floral notes. A surprise came in the form of black peppercorns, which offered a welcome subtle bite. For a more intense taste, briefly toasting the spices revitalized and intensified their flavors. To round out the spices, orange zest (without any bitter pith) gave our mulled drink a fruity essence that brought all the flavors together. Use a heavy saucepan to break the cinnamon stick into pieces. This recipe can easily be doubled in a Dutch oven.

1. Toast cinnamon stick, peppercorns, coriander seeds, and cloves in large saucepan over medium heat, shaking saucepan occasionally, until fragrant, 1 to 3 minutes. Stir in cider and orange zest, bring to simmer, and cook until flavors meld, about 30 minutes. Use wide, shallow spoon to skim off any foam that rises to surface while simmering.

2. Strain cider into serving mugs, discarding solids. Serve. (Strained cider can be refrigerated for up to 1 week. Reheat in large saucepan over medium heat to serve.)

old-fashioned mulled cider

SERVES 6 TO 8

1 **cinnamon stick, broken into pieces**

½ **teaspoon black peppercorns**

½ **teaspoon coriander seeds**

7 **whole cloves**

8 **cups apple cider**

4 **(2-inch) strips orange zest**

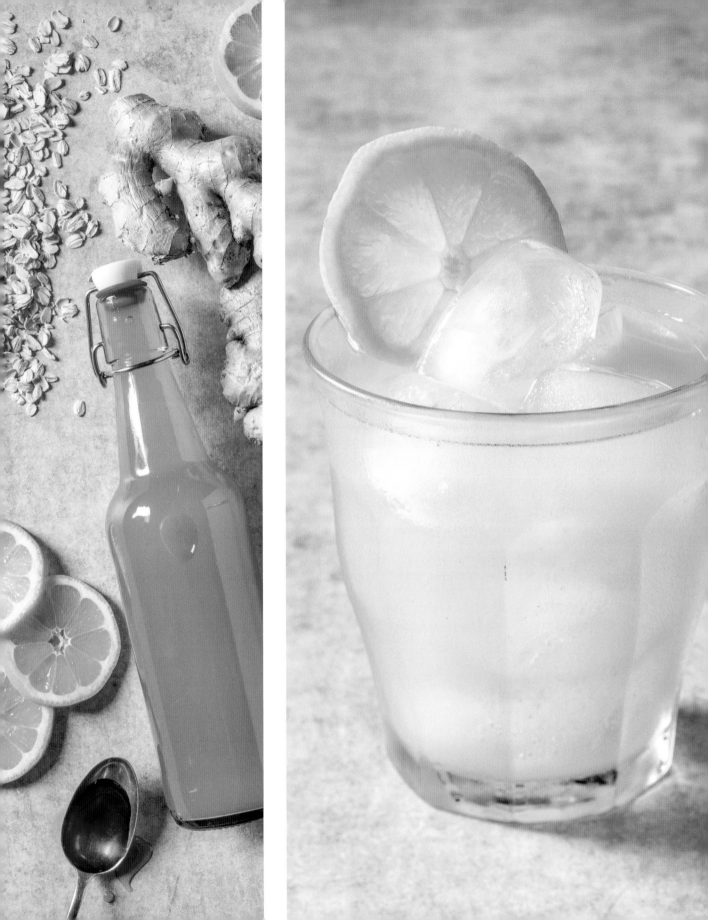

why this combination works: You could consider switchel to be the original energy drink or health tonic, since both cider vinegar and maple syrup contain potassium, an electrolyte, and ginger contains curcumin, which is an anti-inflammatory. Dating back to colonial America, this beverage is all about quenching thirst and fortifying the body for more work. Traditionally served to farmers working in the fields during haying season, it is sometimes referred to as "haymaker's punch" and is still served in some Amish communities. The ginger was a way to quell any stomach issues that might emerge as farmers drank so much water in the fields, and the vinegar helped maintain the balance of acidity already present in the body. We liked the balance of ¾ cup cider vinegar to ½ cup maple syrup. Two tablespoons of grated fresh ginger gave the spicy warmth we were looking for without over-powering the delicate maple flavor. Last but not least, some rolled oats provided hearty body. The longer you let the switchel chill before straining, the stronger the ginger flavor will be. Feel free to adjust the tartness with water to suit your taste.

1. Bring all ingredients to brief simmer in large saucepan over medium-high heat. Let cool to room temperature, about 1 hour. Transfer switchel to bowl, cover, and refrigerate until flavors meld, at least 6 hours or up to 1 day.

2. Strain mixture through fine-mesh strainer set over serving pitcher or large container, pressing on solids to extract as much liquid as possible; discard solids. Serve in chilled old-fashioned glasses or Mason jars filled with ice, garnishing individual portions with lemon slice.

switchel

SERVES 6 TO 8

6 **cups water**

¾ **cup cider vinegar**

½ **cup pure maple syrup**

¼ **cup old-fashioned rolled oats**

2 **tablespoons grated fresh ginger**

1 **teaspoon grated lemon zest, plus lemon slices for garnish**

¼ **teaspoon table salt**

horchata

SERVES 4 TO 6

4½ cups water

1¼ cups whole blanched almonds

¼ cup sugar

⅓ cup long-grain white rice

1½ teaspoons vanilla extract

1 teaspoon ground cinnamon

¼ teaspoon table salt

1 cup evaporated milk

IF YOU DON'T HAVE

whole blanched almonds: Use slivered or sliced almonds.

why this combination works: Every household and restaurant in Mexico boasts its own version of wildly popular horchata, a milky, dessert-like drink made by steeping rice, and sometimes various nuts or seeds, in water with spices, then blending the mixture to creamy goodness. It's the perfect complement to spicy Mexican cuisine or fantastic on its own as a refreshing hot weather treat. While trying different recipes for horchata, we found that adding almonds to the rice base lent more complex flavor and a creamier feel to the beverage. We combined water, sugar, vanilla, cinnamon, and a pinch of salt with the almonds and rice. Letting the mixture soak overnight not only softened the nuts and rice (making blending easier) but also deepened the flavor infusion from the spices. We then blended the mixture until the rice and almonds broke down. The addition of evaporated milk helped make the horchata even creamier.

1. In large bowl, combine water, almonds, sugar, rice, vanilla, cinnamon, and salt. Cover with plastic wrap and let steep at room temperature for at least 12 hours or up to 24 hours.

2. Line fine-mesh strainer with triple layer of cheesecloth overhanging edges; set aside. Process almond mixture in blender until smooth, 30 to 60 seconds. Strain blended almond mixture through prepared strainer into large bowl; discard solids. Pour strained almond liquid into pitcher or storage container. Stir in evaporated milk until well combined. (Horchata can be refrigerated for up to 3 days.) Serve in ice-filled glasses.

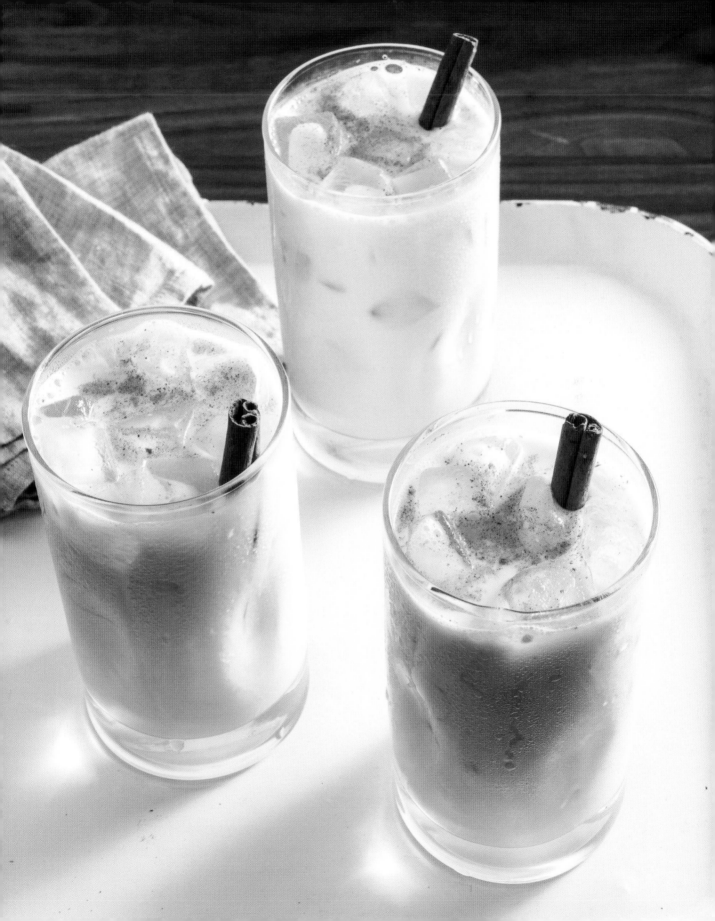

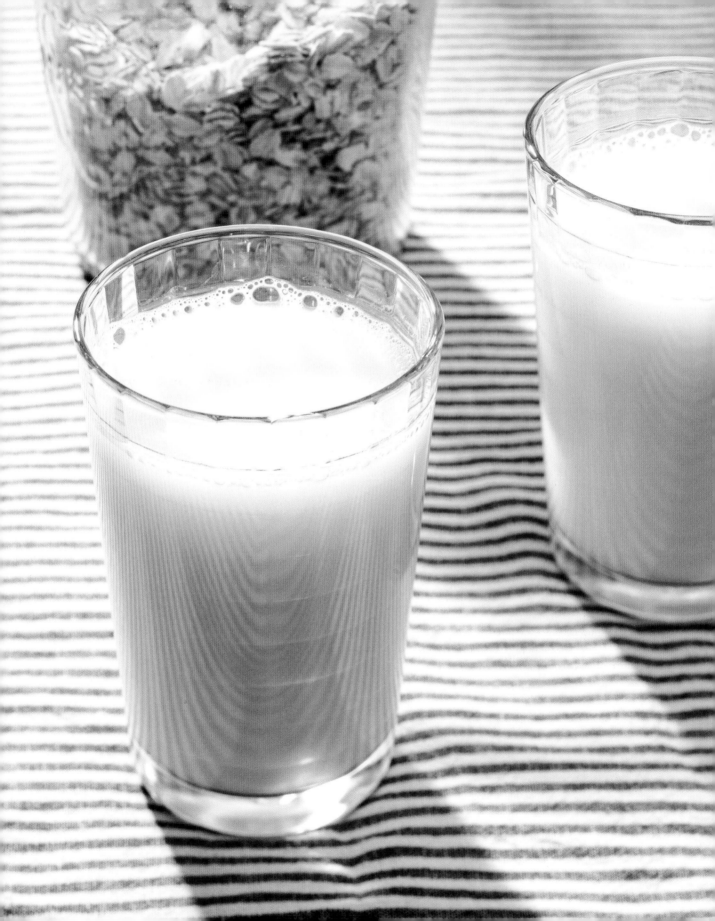

why this combination works: Making your own oat milk is super simple and also inexpensive. We love keeping it on hand to add to smoothies, to bake with, or to just drink straight from the fridge. Oat milk is great if you have sensitivities to soy or nuts, or if you're just trying to avoid animal products. While it may sound intimidating, the entire process of making oat milk is as easy as blending everything together and then straining. To make this recipe customizable, the sugar is optional, so you can have your milk as sweet or neutral as you like. The addition of vegetable oil was crucial to this recipe because it added desired fat and provided a thick and smooth texture. It also helped reduce the amount of foam that forms while processing; do not omit it. Avoid squeezing the oat pulp too firmly; it will cause the milk to be starchy. We found that sugar and vanilla helped round out the flavor for drinking; however, if you're cooking with this milk, we recommend omitting them.

Line fine-mesh strainer with triple layer of cheesecloth overhanging edges; set aside. Process water, oats, sugar (if using), oil, vanilla (if using), and salt in blender until coarsely ground, about 10 seconds, scraping down sides of blender jar as needed. Strain blended oat mixture through prepared strainer into 4-cup liquid measuring cup or large bowl, stirring occasionally, until liquid no longer runs freely, about 5 minutes. Pull edges of cheesecloth together and firmly squeeze pulp until liquid no longer runs freely; discard pulp. Transfer milk to airtight container and refrigerate until well chilled, about 1 hour. Serve. (Oat milk can be refrigerated for up to 4 days; stir to recombine before serving.)

VARIATION
ginger and turmeric oat milk
Add 1 teaspoon grated fresh ginger and ¼ teaspoon ground turmeric to blender with other ingredients.

oat milk

SERVES 4
(MAKES ABOUT 4 CUPS)

- 4 **cups water**
- ¾ **cup old-fashioned rolled oats**
- 2 **teaspoons sugar (optional)**
- ¾ **teaspoon vegetable oil**
- ½ **teaspoon vanilla extract (optional)**
- ⅛ **teaspoon table salt**

IF YOU DON'T HAVE

old-fashioned rolled oats: Use quick-cooking rolled oats.

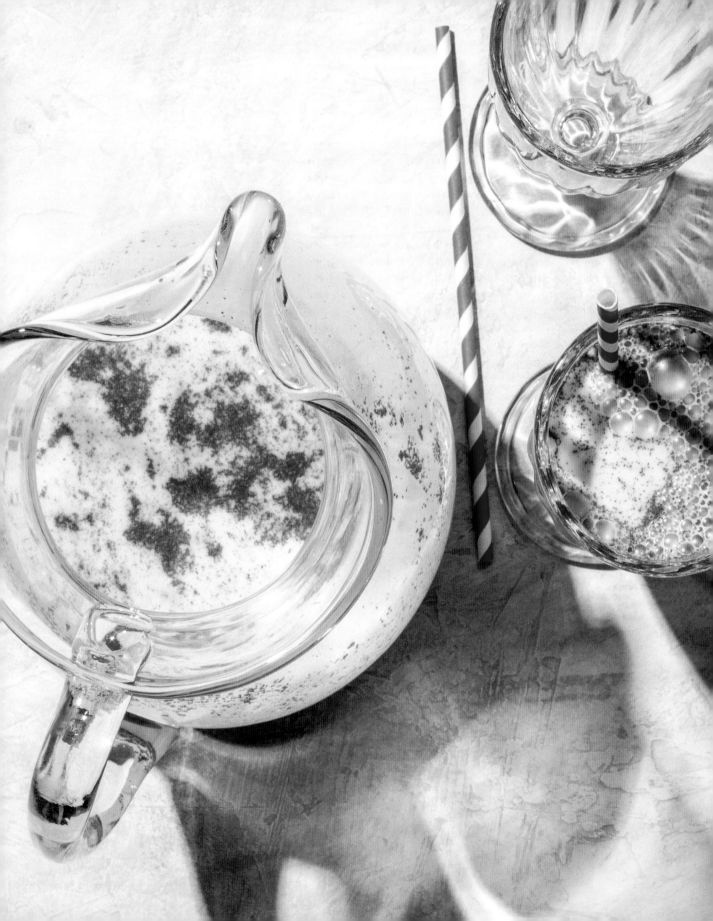

why this combination works: Almond milk is a nutty, creamy, and refreshing dairy-free alternative to animal milk that is beyond easy to make at home. Since many store-bought varieties include thickeners, stabilizers, and gums, we wanted to make our own. While many homemade almond milk recipes require soaking the almonds for at least 8 hours or up to a full day, we skipped soaking altogether in favor of slow cooking in a saucepan. After 2 to 3 hours, we simply drained the almonds, processed them with fresh water in a blender (4 cups of water gave our milk the best flavor and texture), and then poured the mixture through a cheesecloth-lined fine-mesh strainer to separate the milk from the pulp. Since the pulp still contained a great deal of milk, we squeezed it in the cheesecloth until no liquid remained. We found that a hint of salt and a little bit of sugar helped round out the drink and give the milk a subtle sweetness; however, if you plan to cook with this milk, we recommend omitting the sugar.

1. Place almonds in large saucepan and add water to cover by 1 inch. Bring to simmer and cook until almonds are softened, 2 to 3 hours. (Alternatively, place almonds and water in slow cooker, cover, and cook on low for 2 to 3 hours.) Drain almonds and rinse well.

2. Line fine-mesh strainer with triple layer of cheesecloth over-hanging edges; set aside. Process almonds and 4 cups cold water in blender until almonds are finely ground, about 2 minutes. Strain blended almond mixture through prepared strainer into 4-cup liquid measuring cup or large bowl and press to extract as much liquid as possible. Pull edges of cheesecloth together and firmly squeeze pulp until liquid no longer runs freely; discard pulp. Stir in sugar (if using) and salt until completely dissolved. Transfer milk to airtight container and refrigerate until well chilled, about 1 hour. Serve. (Almond milk can be refrigerated for up to 4 days; stir to recombine before serving.)

VARIATION
vanilla-spiced almond milk
Stir 1 teaspoon vanilla extract and 1 teaspoon ground cinnamon into almond milk with salt.

almond milk

SERVES 4
(MAKES ABOUT 4 CUPS)

1¼ cups whole blanched almonds

2 tablespoons sugar (optional)

⅛ teaspoon table salt

IF YOU DON'T HAVE

whole blanched almonds: Use whole raw almonds.

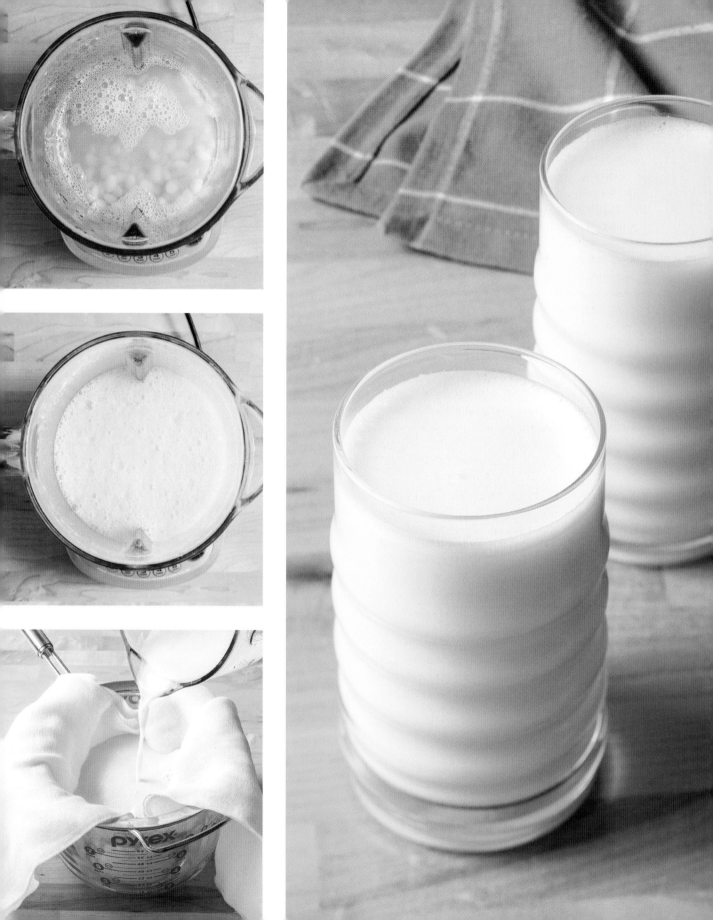

why this combination works: Soy milk is as creamy and rich as almond or oat milk but has a more neutral flavor than either of those for more versatile applications. We think our soy milk is far superior to store-bought because it's made with only four simple ingredients, two of which are optional. Homemade soy milk is also a good source of protein. Our base is made from dried soybeans that we rehydrated. During testing, we discovered that the longer the soybeans soaked, the richer the milk was. After soaking, we combined the rehydrated beans with water and simmered until the beans were tender enough for blending. Straining the blended liquid ensured that our soy milk had a desirable, smooth texture. Soybeans are a good source of plant-based protein, and dried ones are available in well-stocked supermarkets, at Asian markets, and online. We found that sugar and vanilla helped round out the flavor; however, if you're cooking with this milk, we recommend omitting them.

1. Place soybeans in bowl and add water to cover by 2 inches. Soak soybeans at room temperature for at least 1 hour or up to 24 hours. Drain and rinse well.

2. Bring soaked soybeans and 4½ cups water to simmer in medium saucepan. Partially cover and simmer over medium-low heat until soybeans are tender, 30 to 40 minutes.

3. Line fine-mesh strainer with triple layer of cheesecloth over-hanging edges; set aside. Carefully transfer soybeans and cooking liquid to blender. Add sugar (if using), vanilla (if using), and salt and process until mostly smooth, about 3 minutes. Strain blended soybean mixture through prepared strainer into 4-cup liquid measuring cup or large bowl, stirring occasionally, until liquid no longer runs freely and mixture is cool enough to touch, about 30 minutes. Pull edges of cheesecloth together and firmly squeeze pulp until liquid no longer runs freely; discard pulp. Transfer milk to airtight container and refrigerate until well chilled, about 1 hour. Serve. (Soy milk can be refrigerated for up to 4 days; stir to recombine before serving.)

soy milk

SERVES 4
(MAKES ABOUT 4 CUPS)

- ½ **cup dried soybeans, picked over and rinsed**
- 2 **teaspoons sugar (optional)**
- ½ **teaspoon vanilla extract (optional)**
- ⅛ **teaspoon table salt**

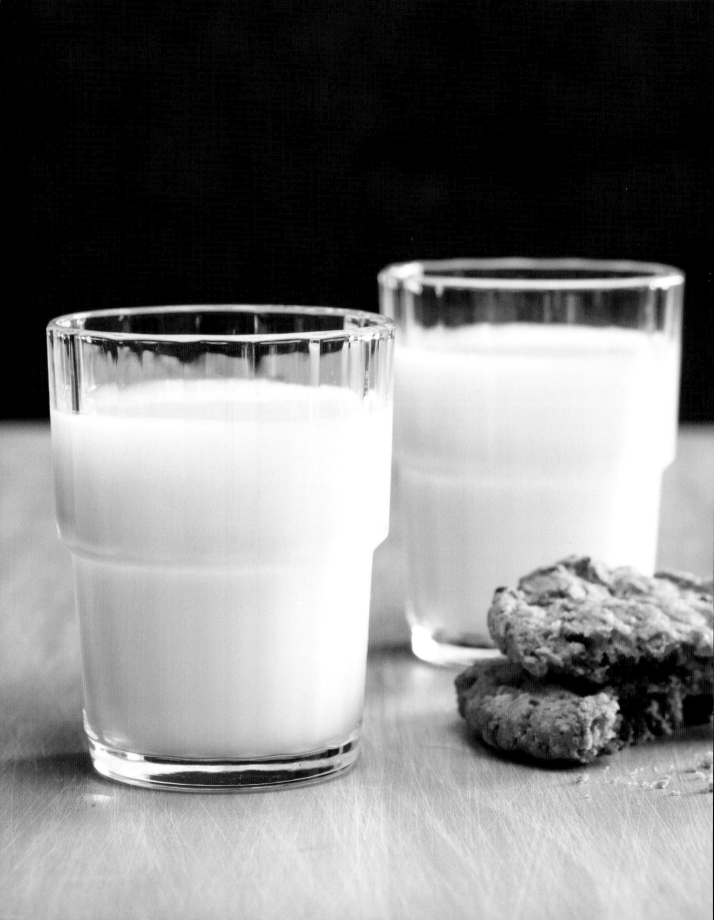

why this combination works: Commercial rice milk is usually too thin and watery to make use of in cooking, but our version is rich-tasting and easy to prepare. We discovered that how you handle the rice matters. We first tried using soaked rice, but the milk was too thick and tasted cooked. After much testing, we found that there was no need to presoak the rice and that we needed far less than expected. Instead of soaking, we simply simmered the rice over low heat for 12 minutes to turn it tender. Blending the rice with all the other ingredients delivered a milk with a creamy texture and fresh flavor. The blender pureed everything, but we strained the milk just in case a few granules were left behind. The oil helps reduce the amount of foam that forms while processing; do not omit it. We found that sugar and vanilla helped round out the flavor; however, if you're cooking with this milk, we recommend omitting them.

1. Bring water, rice, sugar (if using), oil, vanilla (if using), and salt to simmer in large saucepan. Cover and simmer over low heat until rice is very tender, about 12 minutes.

2. Carefully transfer rice mixture to blender and process until opaque and smooth, about 1 minute. Strain blended rice mixture through fine-mesh strainer into 4-cup liquid measuring cup or large bowl, stirring to extract as much liquid as possible; discard solids. Let cool to room temperature, about 30 minutes. Transfer milk to airtight container and refrigerate until well chilled, about 1 hour. Serve. (Rice milk can be refrigerated for up to 4 days; stir to recombine before serving.)

VARIATION
brown rice milk
Substitute long-grain brown rice for white rice and increase simmering time to about 25 minutes.

rice milk

SERVES 4
(MAKES ABOUT 4 CUPS)

4 cups water

2 tablespoons long-grain white rice, rinsed

2 teaspoons sugar (optional)

¾ teaspoon vegetable oil

½ teaspoon vanilla extract (optional)

⅛ teaspoon table salt

chicken broth

MAKES ABOUT 8 CUPS

1 tablespoon extra-virgin olive oil

3 pounds whole chicken legs, backs, and/or wings, hacked into 2-inch pieces

1 onion, chopped

8 cups water, divided

3 bay leaves

1 teaspoon kosher salt

IF YOU DON'T HAVE

bay leaves: Use sage leaves or 2 rosemary sprigs.

why this combination works: This rich and well-rounded chicken broth is perfect for sipping when you want a savory, protein-rich drink, or it can be used in a wide range of cooking applications. Many recipes for chicken broth call for simmering a whole chicken, but we found that cutting the chicken into pieces yielded more flavor by providing more surface area for browning to eke out more flavor, especially from the bone marrow. We tested a variety of vegetables to round out our broth and found that onion enhanced the chicken flavor while also imparting a gentle sweetness. Chopping and then sautéing the onion in chicken fat helped concentrate the onion's flavor. We simmered pots of broth from 1 to 24 hours, and tasters agreed that at 4 hours, our broth had the best flavor—a deep, well-balanced chicken base with a slightly aromatic sweetness. If using a slow cooker, you will need one that holds 5½ to 7 quarts.

1. Heat oil in Dutch oven over medium-high heat until just smoking. Pat chicken dry with paper towels. Brown half of chicken, about 5 minutes; transfer to large bowl. Repeat with remaining chicken; transfer to bowl.

2. Add onion to fat left in pot and cook over medium heat until softened, about 5 minutes. Stir in 2 cups water, bay leaves, and salt, scraping up any browned bits.

3a. for stovetop: Stir remaining 6 cups water into pot, then return browned chicken and any accumulated juices to pot and bring to simmer. Reduce heat to low, cover, and simmer gently until broth is flavorful, about 4 hours.

3b. for slow cooker: Transfer browned chicken, accumulated juices, and onion mixture to slow cooker. Stir in remaining 6 cups water. Cover and cook on low until broth is flavorful, about 4 hours.

4. Remove large bones, then strain broth through fine-mesh strainer into large container; discard solids. Let broth settle for 5 to 10 minutes, then defat using wide, shallow spoon or fat separator. Ladle broth into heatproof mugs and serve. (Cooled broth can be refrigerated for up to 4 days or frozen for up to 1 month. To reheat, bring 1 cup broth to simmer in small saucepan.)

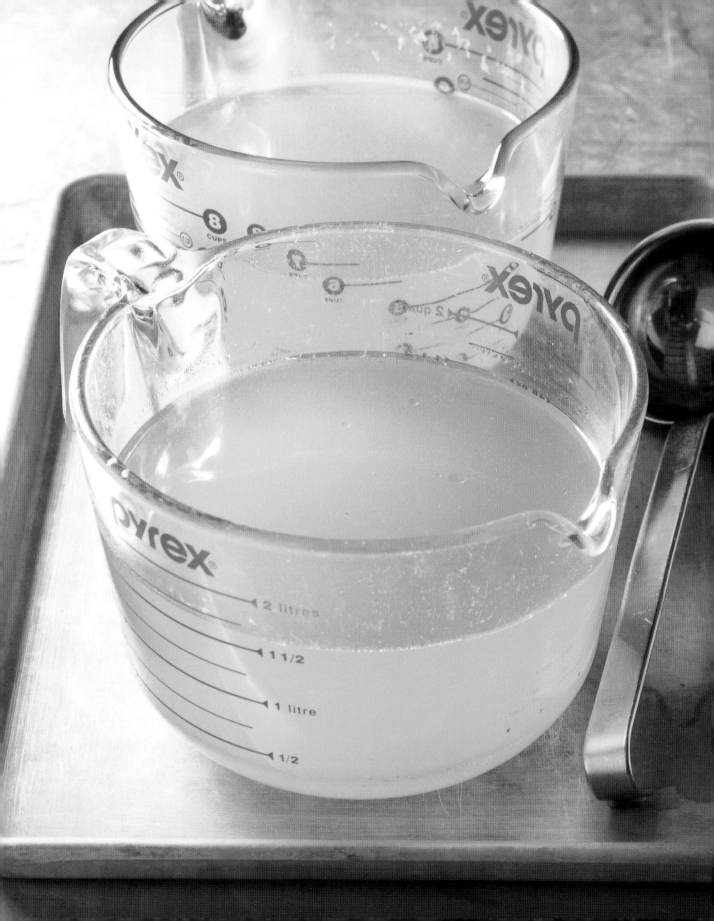

beef broth

MAKES ABOUT 8 CUPS

- 2 **tablespoons extra-virgin olive oil, divided**
- 6 **pounds oxtails**
- 1 **large onion, chopped**
- 8 **ounces white mushrooms, trimmed and chopped**
- 2 **tablespoons tomato paste**
- 10 **cups water, divided**
- 3 **bay leaves**
- 1 **teaspoon kosher salt**
- ¼ **teaspoon pepper**

IF YOU DON'T HAVE

bay leaves: Use sage leaves or 2 rosemary sprigs.

why this combination works: We set out to create a flavorful, nuanced beef broth that could be enjoyed as a drink to add protein and nutrients to your day. We used oxtails because they are economical, all-in-one bundles of flavor-packed meat, fat, collagen-rich connective tissue, and bone marrow. Plus, they're sold precut, which reduces prep time. We browned them to create fond, then sautéed an onion and mushrooms in the rendered fat. Tomato paste gave our base extra umami flavor, which resulted in a beautiful deeply colored broth with rich, beefy flavor and a luxurious, silky texture. Buy oxtails that are approximately 2 inches thick and 2 to 4 inches in diameter. Oxtails can often be found in the freezer section of the grocery store; if using frozen oxtails, thaw them completely before using. If using a slow cooker, you will need one that holds 5½ to 7 quarts.

1. Heat 1 tablespoon oil in Dutch oven over medium-high heat until just smoking. Pat oxtails dry with paper towels. Brown half of oxtails, 7 to 10 minutes; transfer to large bowl. Repeat with remaining 1 tablespoon oil and remaining oxtails; transfer to bowl.

2. Add onion and mushrooms to fat left in pot and cook until softened and lightly browned, about 5 minutes. Stir in tomato paste and cook until fragrant, about 1 minute. Stir in 2 cups water, bay leaves, salt, and pepper, scraping up any browned bits.

3a. for oven: Adjust oven rack to middle position and heat oven to 200 degrees. Stir remaining 8 cups water into pot, then return browned oxtails and any accumulated juices to pot and bring to simmer. Fit large piece of aluminum foil over pot, pressing to seal, then cover tightly with lid. Transfer pot to oven and cook until broth is flavorful, about 24 hours.

3b. for slow cooker: Transfer browned oxtails, accumulated juices, and vegetable mixture to slow cooker. Stir in remaining 8 cups water. Cover and cook on low until broth is flavorful, about 24 hours.

4. Remove large bones, then strain broth through fine-mesh strainer into large container; discard solids. Let broth settle for 5 to 10 minutes, then defat using wide, shallow spoon or fat separator. Ladle broth into heat-proof mugs and serve. (Cooled broth can be refrigerated for up to 4 days or frozen for up to 1 month. To reheat, bring 1 cup broth to simmer in small saucepan).

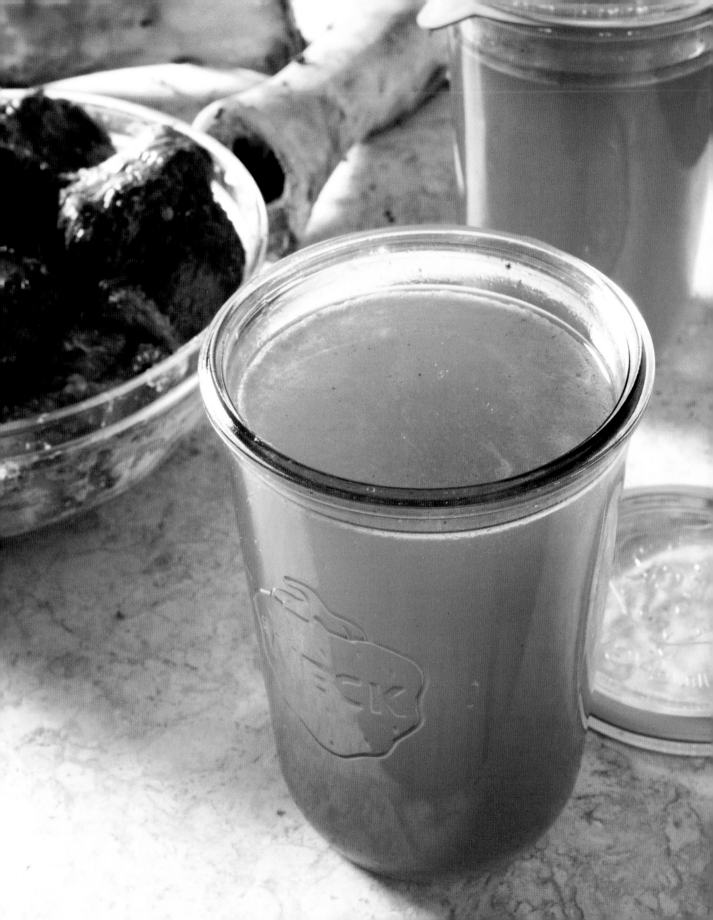

vegetable broth base

MAKES ABOUT 1¾ CUPS BASE

(ENOUGH FOR 7 QUARTS BROTH)

- 2 leeks, white and light-green parts only, chopped and washed thoroughly (2½ cups or 5 ounces)
- ½ small celery root, peeled and cut into ½-inch pieces (¾ cup or 3 ounces)
- 2 carrots, peeled and cut into ½-inch pieces (⅔ cup or 3 ounces)
- ½ cup (½ ounce) fresh parsley leaves and thin stems
- 3 tablespoons dried minced onions
- 2 tablespoons kosher salt
- 1½ tablespoons tomato paste
- 3 tablespoons soy sauce

IF YOU DON'T HAVE

kosher salt: Use 1 tablespoon table salt.

soy sauce: Use coconut aminos.

why this combination works: A good vegetable broth can be the perfect vegetarian option for a sipping broth to start your day or to curb hunger. Unfortunately, supermarket offerings don't taste like fresh vegetables, and homemade versions can be expensive and time-consuming to make. For the simple preparation in our recipe, we processed a selection of fresh vegetables, salt, and savory ingredients to a concentrated paste that we could store in the freezer and reconstitute as needed. Celery root and carrots gave us a traditional base. Leeks provided good allium flavor, and a small amount of dried minced onions supported the fresh flavor of the leeks. Parsley brought a touch of fresh herbal flavor, while tomato paste and soy sauce gave the mix an umami boost. For the best balance of flavors, measure the prepped vegetables by weight. Kosher salt aids in grinding the vegetables and keeps the broth from freezing solid, making it easy to remove 1 tablespoon at a time.

1. Process leeks, celery root, carrots, parsley, dried onions, and salt in food processor, scraping down sides of bowl frequently, until paste is as fine as possible, 3 to 4 minutes. Add tomato paste and process for 1 minute, scraping down sides of bowl every 20 seconds. Add soy sauce and continue to process for 1 minute.

2. Transfer mixture to airtight container and tap firmly on counter to remove air bubbles. Press small piece of parchment paper flush against surface of mixture and cover. (Base can be frozen for up to 6 months.)

3. to make 1 cup broth: Stir 1 tablespoon fresh or frozen broth base into 1 cup boiling water. If particle-free broth is desired, let broth steep for 5 minutes, then strain through fine-mesh strainer.

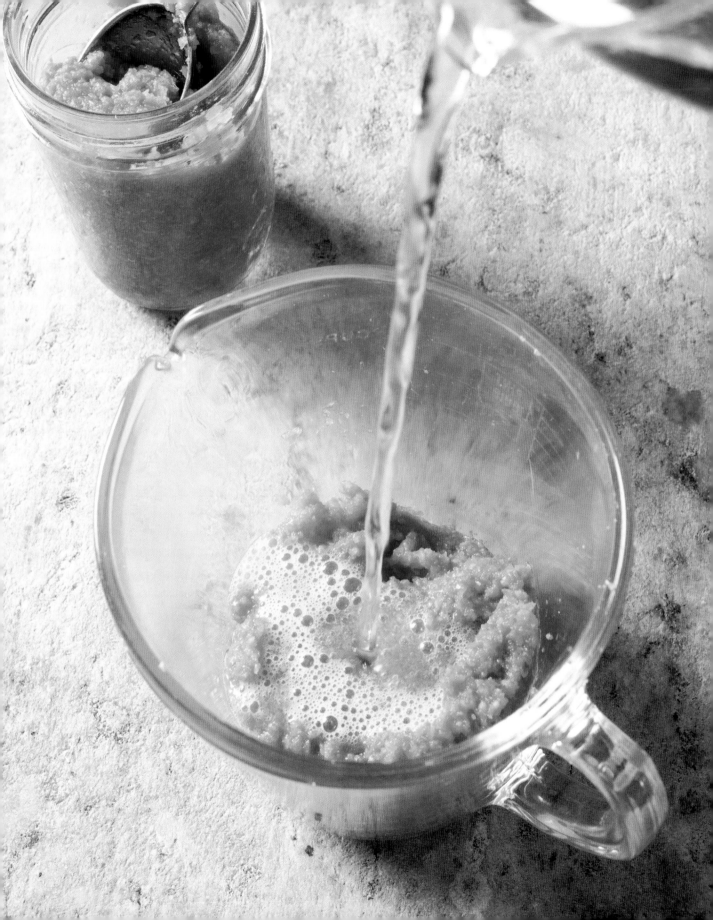

conversions and equivalents

Some say cooking is a science and an art. We would say that geography has a hand in it, too. Flours and sugars manufactured in the United Kingdom and elsewhere will feel and taste different from those manufactured in the United States. So we cannot promise that the loaf of bread you bake in Canada or England will taste the same as a loaf baked in the States, but we can offer guidelines for converting weights and measures. We also recommend that you rely on your instincts when making our recipes. Refer to the visual cues provided.

The recipes in this book were developed using standard U.S. measures following U.S. government guidelines. The charts below offer equivalents for U.S. and metric measures. All conversions are approximate and have been rounded up or down to the nearest whole number.

EXAMPLE

1 teaspoon = 4.9292 milliliters, rounded up to 5 milliliters
1 ounce = 28.3495 grams, rounded down to 28 grams

CONVERTING FAHRENHEIT TO CELSIUS

We include temperatures in some of the recipes in this book and we recommend an instant-read thermometer for the job. To convert Fahrenheit degrees to Celsius, use this simple formula:

Subtract 32 degrees from the Fahrenheit reading, then divide the result by 1.8 to find the Celsius reading. For example, to convert 160°F to Celsius:

160°F − 32 = 128°
128° ÷ 1.8 = 71.11°C, rounded down to 71°C

VOLUME CONVERSIONS

U.S.	Metric
1 teaspoon	5 milliliters
2 teaspoons	10 milliliters
1 tablespoon	15 milliliters
2 tablespoons	30 milliliters
¼ cup	59 milliliters
⅓ cup	79 milliliters
½ cup	118 milliliters
¾ cup	177 milliliters
1 cup	237 milliliters
1¼ cups	296 milliliters
1½ cups	355 milliliters
2 cups (1 pint)	473 milliliters
2½ cups	591 milliliters
3 cups	710 milliliters
4 cups (1 quart)	0.946 liter
1.06 quarts	1 liter
4 quarts (1 gallon)	3.8 liters

WEIGHT CONVERSIONS

Ounces	Grams
½	14
¾	21
1	28
1½	43
2	57
2½	71
3	85
3½	99
4	113
4½	128
5	142
6	170
7	198
8	227
9	255
10	283
12	340
16 (1 pound)	454

index

Note: Page references in *italics* indicate photographs.